A Guide To
ALLERGIES

Published by
Lotus Press

A Guide to ALLERGIES

Dr. Ramdass
&
Anuradha Shiva Kumar

Lotus PRESS
4263/3, Ansari Road,
Darya Ganj, New Delhi- 110002

Lotus Press
4263/3, Ansari Road, Darya Ganj, New Delhi-110002
Ph.: 32903912, 23280047, E-mail: lotus_press@sify.com
www.lotuspress.co.in

A Guide to Allergies

ISBN: 81-89093-79-7

Reprint: 2010

Published by: **Lotus Press**, New Delhi-110 002
Printed at: DD Offset Printing Press, Noida.

Contents

PREFACE

This book can be termed as 'A to Z' of Allergy, as the book has almost everything on allergy. It starts with an introduction to allergy and ends in the latest developments in the field of allergy.

This book gives everything that other books on allergy give, i.e., asthma, rhinitis and skin allergies. But the USP of this book lies in the fact that it doesn't stop with the above three. It moves forward and covers:

a) Facts and myths on allergies.

b) Allergic conjunctivitis.

c) Immunotherapy for allergies in detail.

d) Auto allergy diseases with brief notes on blood, cancer, graft immune responses and certain controversial sections.

e) 'Drug rashes' of all kinds and how they differ from drug allergy rashes.

f) Allergy systems of medicine—what are they and what they speak about asthma in their own terms and conditions.

We would like the readers to read this book with three aspects in mind :

1. Give special attention to the 'extra' information on allergy given only in this book.

2. Keep a medical glossary; if any doubt arises refer to it; if certain sections are 'too medical' you can restrict to just a brief study. Getting to know the 'terms' is important as the idea is to know everything, i.e., the A to Z of allergy.

3. If there is 'any' criticism on inclusion of 'migraine' in this book please forgive us and carry on reading the rest of the book.

We would be happy if the readers give us a feedback after reading this book. This book is open to criticism and the purpose of the book would be solved only when it receives both bouquets and brickbats. Bouquets give encouragement to give a better book and brickbats aid in correcting the various shortcomings in the book.

Happy reading!

Dr. Ramdass

Anuradha Shivakumar

1
ALLERGY : INTRODUCTION AND CLASSIFICATION

Allergy : An Introduction

Allergy is a reaction of the body to a harmless substance. Allergies occur when the immune system produces antibodies and sensitised white blood cells when exposed to substances that are normally harmless. When the immune system encounters the substances for the second time, it releases histamine and various other chemicals. These *chemicals* are responsible for the symptoms of allergy such as sneezing, nasal congestion, itchy swelling, inflammation of the eyes, vomiting or narrowing of the airways in asthma. Substances like pollens of the flowers; spores of fungi; house dust, particles of animal hair; food substances like eggs, fish, wheat, nuts; metabolic elements like nickel, chromium; drugs like penicillin and sulpha; rubber and cosmetic products can produce an allergy.

These may be harmless to many people but can trigger off allergic responses in some. Common allergies such as asthma, eczema or hayfever are caused by reactions to substances such as pollen, house dust. Many people also suffer from skin allergies to substances such as rubber or cosmetic products. Food allergies are also fairly common and can be very severe. For example, some sufferers develop fatal reactions to nuts and shellfish. Symptoms of food allergies are diarrhoea, vomiting, abdominal cramps. Metallic elements like nickel, chromium can cause skin reactions.

Penicillin and sulphur drugs can produce anaphylactic reaction in which a patient goes into severe allergic reaction, develops shock and may just collapse.

What is an Allergen ?

The substance causing reaction in an allergic person is called allergen or antigen.

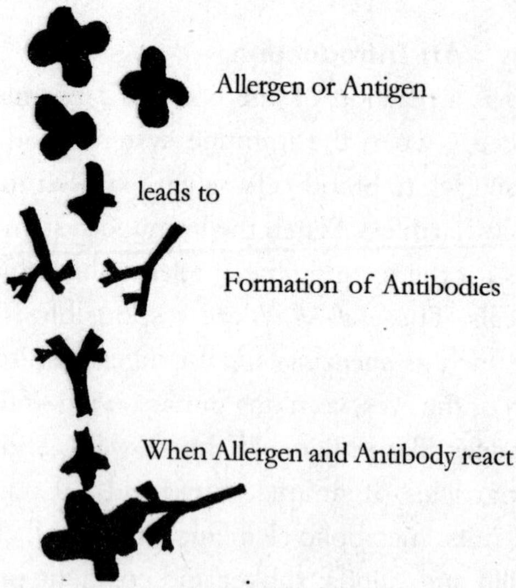

Fig. 1.1 : Antigen-Antibody Complex

What is an antibody ?

The substance which is produced in the body of the allergic person due to introduction of the antigen is called an antibody. When antigen and antibody meet together and react the process is known as Antigen-Antibody reaction.

Antigen-Antibody reactions are of various types. This depends on the (1) nature of the antigen (2) nature of antibodies and (3) various other factors like the mode of introduction of the antigen.

An asthma-prone person has in his blood and organs the antibodies called 'Reagin'. It is a gamma globulin (a protein). This is represented as IGE. (Here we must know that 'Blocking antibodies' and 'Haemagglidinating' antibodies are other forms of antibodies. These like Reagins produce immediate allergic reactions).

IgM, IgD, IgA, IgD—are all other types of antibodies. Each has a specific role. The Ig stands for Immunoglobulin and the letters M, G, A, D and E stand for respective classes of antibodies. For the purpose of our present limited discussion, we shall just learn about a few.

IgE—constitutes only a very small per cent of antibodies and is associated with allergy.

IgG—constitutes 45 per cent of antibodies of the normal person.

IgM—involved in primary responses, i.e., what occurs on first exposure to a specific antigen.

IgE in the blood or organ resides on the surface of a cell called Mast Cell. When an allergen (or antigen) reacts with the IgE present on the surface of mast cell, first the mast cell membrane ruptures and chemicals like histamine, serotonin, eosonophil chemotactic substance, slow reacting substance of anaphylaxis, a protease, a neutrophil chemotactic substance, heparin, platelet activating factors are released. These substances cause such phenomena as :

1) dilatation of local blood vessels.
2) attraction of eosonophills and basophills to reactive site (this is called Chemotaxis).
3) damage to local tissues by protease.
4) increased permeability of capillaries, and loss of fluid into tissues.
5) contraction of local smooth muscle cells.

These processes cause the manifestations of allergy according to the type of tissue in which allergen reagin reaction is taking place such as :

a) Spasm of the muscles of lung airways in asthma.

b) Exudation of fluid from the nasal mucous membrane in cases of seasonal sneezing (hay fever).

c) Swelling, irritation and redness of skin in cases of urticaria. The swellings are called 'hives'.

d) 'Widespread Anaphylaxis' leading to shock, collapse if allergen is injected into circulation directly.

e) Asthma, urticaria, hay fever, seasonal or perennial sneezing, eczema, anaphylaxis are all many and diverse manifestations of one entity called 'Allergy'.

Allergy Facts

GLORIA (Global Resources In Allergy) is the World Allergy Organization's (WAO) flagship education programme that educates medical professionals worldwide through regional presentations and local training programmes. The objective of the GLORIA is to empower doctors with practical skills.

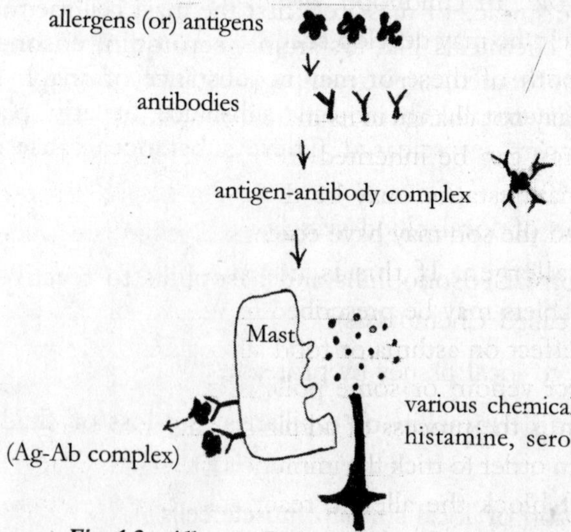

Fig. 1.2 : Allergy : Pathogenesis and Manifestations

These chemicals produce

1) Increased permeability of capillaries
2) Vasodilatation of blood vessels
3) Attraction of various cells (by chemotaxis) to site
4) Damage to local tissues

All these constitute an:

Allergic Reaction → Manifests as

- Irritation Swelling/ Redness of skin → 'Urticaria'
- Spasm of lung muscles airways → Asthma
- Fluid exudation in nasal mucous membrane, sneezing → Hay fever
- Severe shock/ collapse → 'Anaphylaxis'

Allergy can change (in a person) in its manifestation as the person grows old. In childhood, he may have eczema. As he becomes an adult, he may develop sneezing. As he still grows old, he may have both of these or may become asthmatic. On the other hand, it may not change in its manifestation and may remain as it was. Allergy can be inherited from one generation to the next, but its manifestation may be different, like a father may have asthma and the son may have eczema. The best treatment is to avoid the allergen. If this is not possible, a course of antihistamine tablets may be prescribed to relieve the symptoms. They have no effect on asthma or food allergy. Sufferers who are allergic to insect venom or some pollens may be de-sensitised. De-sensitisation is the process of administering, increasing doses of the allergen in order to trick the immune system into producting antibodies that block the allergic reactions. This treatment is successful for two out of three sufferers but may have some side effects such as itching or swelling.

Summary

1) Allergy is a reaction of the body to a harmless substance.
2) Pollens, house dust, food substances, drugs are all common allergens.
3) Allergens trigger the production of antibodies in our body. Allergens (or antigens) and antibody complex initiate allergic reaction through a cascade of events involving chemicals released from mast cells.
4) Manifestations of allergic reaction are diverse.
5) Asthma, hay fever, urticaria are all allergic conditions.
6) Avoiding the allergen, antihistamines, desensitisation are three important treatment modalities for allergies.

Allergic Reactions : Classification

It is customary to apply the term allergy to all manifestations of increased sensitivity induced in the organism by the reaction of allergens (antigens) with antibodies. The clinical symptoms of allergy are extremely varied.

Allergic reactions are of two main types:

1) allergic reactions of the immediate type.

2) allergic reactions of the delayed type.

Rapid development is a common property of all forms of immediate type of allergy. A cutaneous (skin) allergic reaction of the immediate type develops within several minutes following intracutaneous infection of allergen. This group of immediate type allergic reaction includes :

1) anaphylaxis
2) serum sickness
3) allergic bronchial asthma
4) pollinoses (hay fever)
5) urticaria
6) allergic reactions pertaining to haemorrhagic phenomena.

In allergies of the delayed type, the reaction occurs many hours after exposure to the allergen. This group of delayed type of allergic reactions consists of :

1) Tuberculin type reaction (bacterial allergy)
2) Contact type reactions (contact dermatitis)
3) Auto allergic or auto immune reactions; this includes encephalitis, thyroiditis, orchitis, myocarditis, etc.)
4) Allergic reactions of graft rejection
5) Allergic reactions to purified proteins.

ADO's Pathogenic classification of allergic reactions classifies allergic reactions as systemic and local (organ, tissue). These are further classified as chimergic (immediate), kitergic (cell delayed) and so on. These are all beyond the scope of this book and hence will not be discussed in detail.

2

ASTHMA : DEFINITION TO DIFFERENT DIAGNOSIS

Asthma is difficulty in breathing due to narrowing of the small airways in lungs called the bronchioles. Bronchial asthma commonly called asthma consists of repeated attacks of breathlessness and wheezing. Most doctors would agree that asthma is on the increase probably due to rising levels of pollution. Some estimates put the number of sufferers in the UK as high as several million though most of these cases will be mild. In India, asthma cases are on a steady rise. *Hospital Statistics* indicates that asthma has increased over the years in both the out-patient wards and has also become an important and frequent case in emergency wards and admission wards.

When the patient is not in an attack, he feels normal, but when he comes in contact with an allergic substance, it acts as an 'allergen' and this allergen (antigen) reacts with specific antibodies present already in his body. Chemical substances like histamine, and other substances are liberated which produce various allergic reactions inducing the following changes in the bronchi of lungs (1) bronchial muscles under go a constriction which narrows their diameter (2) mucous membrane of the bronchi gets swollen; secretions are poured from this swollen mucous membrane. All these further narrow the lumen of the bronchi.

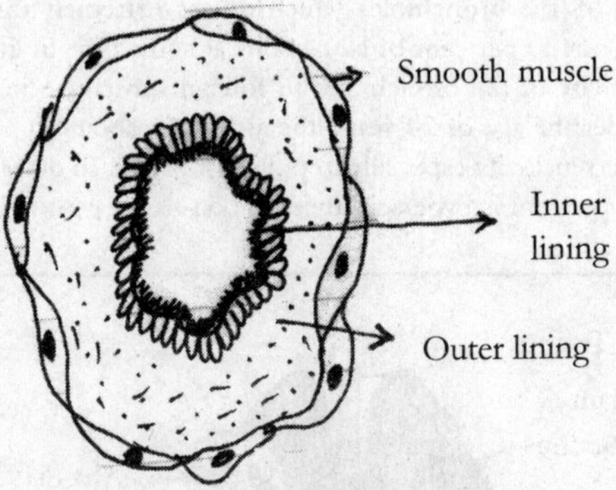

Fig. 2.1 : Normal Bronchus

The diagram above shows the cross section of a normal bronchial tube. Now let us see what happens to the lumen when there is an attack of asthma.

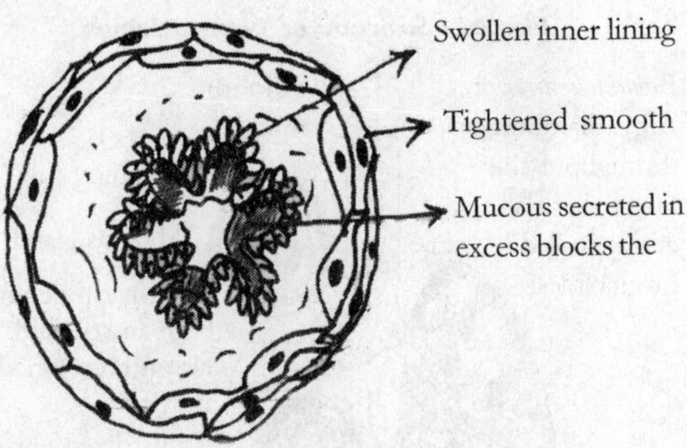

Fig. 2.2 : Constricted Bronchus during an Attack of Asthma

When the bronchi are constricted and are filled with secretions, the patient has difficulty in breathing and there is a wheezing sound in it. When he breathes out, this wheezing increases as the bronchi get narrower.

Medical books describe asthma as a condition that is characterised by spastic contraction of the bronchioles which causes extremely difficult breathing. It occurs in about 30 per cent of all persons at some time in life. The usual case is hyperseshsitivity of the bronchioles to foreign substances in the air. In younger patients under the age of 30 years, the asthma in about 70 per cent is caused by allergic hypersensitivity especially to pollen of plants. In older persons, the causes in about 10 per cent is hypersensitivity to non-allergic types of irritants in the air such as irritants in smog.

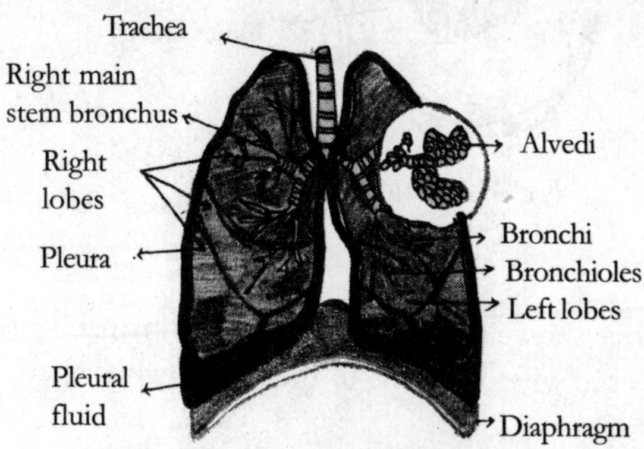

Fig. 2.3 : Structure of Normal Lungs

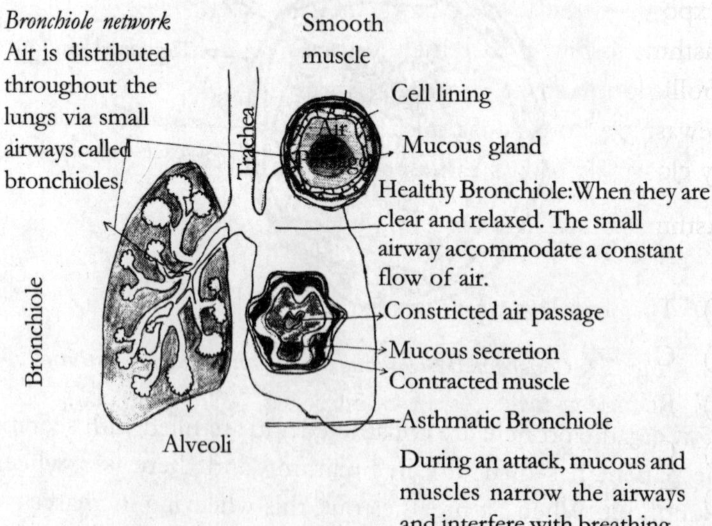

Fig. 2.4 : Anatomy of an Asthma Attack

When the respiration system is working properly, the air we breathe passes in and out of the lungs through a network of airways. But for people with asthma even a minor irritant will set off an immune response that can shut down the airways.

Asthma is a disease of the larger and medium-sized airways of the lungs, and there is obstruction to outflow of air from lungs. Since there is not enough air reaching the lungs for gas exchange, there is *hyper ventilation*, i.e., hurried breathing to compensate. Asthmatic persons usually can inspire quite adequately but have great difficulty expiring. This is the cause for 'dyspnoea' or Air Hunger. Over a long period of time, the chest cage becomes permanently enlarged causing a *barrel chest.* Cough is a frequent symptom in asthmatics. This is more prominent if there is also an infection. Cough is mainly to throw out the excess secretions formed in lungs. The airways of the asthmatics are hyper-reactive to various substances like pollutants in air, pollens, changes in temperature, exercise or physical strains and stress. When they are exposed to the above factors, they react strongly. Persons who are asthmatic find it extremely difficult to tolerate smoking and air pollution. Smoke or strong fumes, smells of fresh paint, whitewashing, house dust, dust from old books and files, opening dusty closets or rooms can all cause severe symptoms in them.

Asthma patients are susceptible to various complications, such as :

1) Thoracic deformity in children
2) Growth retardation
3) Recurrent infection or pneumonia
4) Chronic bronchitis
5) Emphysema—'Excess air in lungs'. This is a chronic and complex destructive process of lungs leading to hyper-inflation of lung tissues.

'Asthma Facts' : In Pregnancy

Uncontrolled asthma can:

Decrease oxygen in foetal blood, possibly impairing foetal growth and survival.

Types of Asthma

Bronchial asthma is classified on the basis of the causative factor. It is classified basically into two major types :

Extrinsic Asthma   Intrinsic Asthma

Extrinsic asthma: is caused by allergic reaction to exposed allergens, the most common allergens being pollens, house dust, fungal spores. These patients often present other allergic manifestations like rhinitis, eczema, etc. They benefit from anti- allergic treatments. This type of asthma occurs in early period of life.

Intrinisic asthma The patients do not have any allergic history, but develop the disease due to some pre-existing disease or infections of the lung. This type of asthma is often seen in persons suffering from chronic bronchitis. Intrinsic asthma does not respond to anti-allergic treatments and occurs (unlike extrinsic asthma) in later period of life.

Exercise-induced asthma is a condition occurring in some individuals after they take a physical exercise or workout. This occurs when workouts are done in cold weather.

Differential Diagnosis of Asthma

We must be able to differentiate asthma from certain conditions that resemble it. In elderly persons, it becomes a difficulty when one has to differentiate between bronchitis and emphysema. Asthma can also co-exist with chronic bronchitis. A patient may begin with asthma because of an allergy to pollens but if not treated may proceed to develop chronic bronchitis and emphysema or later this may lead to intrinsic Asthma and emphysema often. Which is primary and which is secondary is difficult to distinguish.

Bronchitis is a sudden or continuous infection which blocks the airways of the lungs. Bronchitis is a good example of an illness that means different things to different people. Medicos describe it as an "Inflammation of the Bronchus'. In plain language, this means irritation of the larger air passages. Doctors often describe it as an acute/chronic infection in the lungs. To the patient bronchitis can often simply mean an "irritating cough".

Causes of Bronchitis

It is mainly due to an infection. Viruses are the most common causative agents. If there is severe cough, wheeze, especially at nights, one may have to consult a doctor. Virus can bring in a secondary bacterial infection. Cough can become 'productive' (coloured phlegm is brought up by coughing—this is the characteristic 'bronchial cough'). Cold weather, smoke, pollutants in atmosphere can all cause/prolong coughs. *Cigarette smoking is probably the most common cause of bronchitis in the adult population.*

If an allergy triggers a Bronchitis, it is called asthma. The smoker's cough is one form of bronchitis that is all too familiar to doctors. The patient usually is in his 30's and complains of shortness of breath. This and the production of phlegm have gone on for so long that the patient has accepted it as normal. Unless smoking is stopped at once, the acute condition inevitably deteriorates into chronic bronchitis or severe breathlessness.

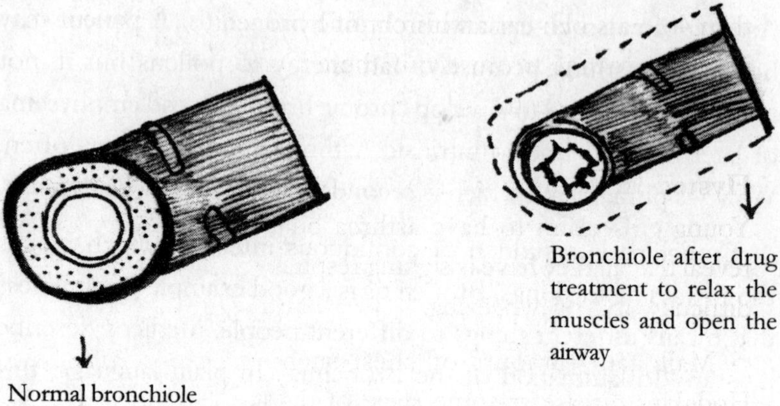

Fig. 2.5 : Cross section of Branchioles

Treatment

Most cases of bronchitis can be treated at home. A regular intake of fluids including honey, lemon or even a little alcohol at night will provide some soothing relief. Also recommended is a sharp intake of some moisture in the form of steam just before the patient goes to bed. The patient can also try sleeping with an extra pillow. If the cough persists or breathing becomes difficult, the doctor prescribes a course of antibiotics or a drug that will relax the muscles and open up the airways and make breathing easier. (See diagram)

Cardiac Asthma

Cardiac asthma is caused by fluid accumulating in the lungs, making it difficult to breathe. This usually happens when the pumping action of the left side of the heart is reduced, resulting in congestion and increased pressure in the blood circulation through the lungs. It is usually a result of old age and can be caused by taking beta blockers. The sufferer may be treated for heart failure with broncho dilator drugs. Cardiac asthma stimulates bronchiol asthma. It should be suspected if the patient is more than 40 years old; has an history of hypertension or heart disease; if he is sweating profusely; if there is air hunger; and he has a sudden fear of death.

Hysterical Asthma

Young girls claim to have asthma but history and examination reveal that all they have is sighing respiration. There is no breathing difficulty and no wheezing.

Malignant tumours of chest such as lymphosarcoma and Hodgkins disease at some stage of disease can mimic bronchial asthma. In bronchogenic carcinoma (lung cancer) '*pressure effect*', i.e., pressure due to enlarged glands in lung, can cause wheezing and breathlessness. Aortic aneurysm (dilated aorta in chest can also cause this. Aorta is the major blood vessel in our body and carries pure oxygenated blood from the heart to the different parts of the body. Some of the diseases caused by inhalation of different types of dusts, vegetative and non-vegetative (organic and inorganic) can give rise to symptoms akin to bronchial asthma. Referred to as '*occupational asthma*' it is stimulated by fumes (epoxy resins, plastics); organic and chemical dusts (wood, cotton, platinum); gases (toluene) and other chemicals (formaldehyde, penicillin).

Some critics mention a 'mixed' type in which there is a mixed pattern and has both intrinsic and extrinsic factors operating in causing the pathology. Some critics go into detail and classify asthma on the basis of principal stimuli that provoke the attacks. Though it is beyond the scope of this book we will just follow it through a table as given in the next page:

Table 2.1 : Types of Asthma and Precipitating Factors

Types of Asthma	*Precipitating Factors**		*Mechanism*
1) Atopic (allergic)	Specific allergens	—	Immune reaction, i.e., antigen, anti-body reaction
2) Non-reaginic	Respiratory tract infection	—	Unknown hyper-active airways
3) Pharmacologic (aspirin sensitive)	Aspirin	—	Certain decrease and increase of local chemicals
4) Occupational	Chemical challenges	—	Immune reaction
5) Allergic broncho-pulmonary aspergillosis	Spores of fungus 'Aspergillus'	—	Immune reaction

* all types may be precipitated by cold, stress, exercise.

Summary

1) Asthma is difficulty in breathing due to narrowing of the small airways in lungs.
2) Bronchial asthma commonly called asthma consists of repeated attacks of breathlessness and wheezing.
3) Asthma is basically divided into two types:
   a) Extrinsic (Allergic type)
   b) Intrinsic (Non-allergic type)
4) Asthma, classified on the basis of precipitating factors, includes two main types :
   a) Aspirin-induced
   b) Occupational type
5) Certain conditions like bronchitis, cardiac asthma, hysterical asthma are the differential diagnosis for bronchial asthma. History, physical examination, signs of symptoms can easily distinguish the two entities.

3

EXTRINSIC ASTHMA : CAUSES

Some Interesting Facts on Allergens

Allergens are not harmful invaders. They are present either in our surroundings or in our food. We are all exposed to them and nothing happens as long as the immunity is normal. The commonest allergens are the inhalants or airborne allergens. House dust is one most complained of. It is a complex substance containing organic and inorganic material. The older the house dust, more allergic it is the meaning thereby that it contains a viable material, the concentration of which increases on storage. A tiny insect called the dust mite is a major allergenic component of house dust. These mites feed on the skin scales shed by humans and pets, and multiply rapidly in humid and dark places. They live, forage, make love, multiply and die in beds, sofas, carpets, rugs, curtains and collected dust. Body parts of the mites, faecel pellets become virulent airborne allergens that are never seen by the naked eye but only perceived by the allergy sufferers through their symptoms.

Insects, like cockroaches, cause allergy when their droppings, urinary droplets or live parts become airborne allergens. Fungal spores are present both inside and outside. They get easily cultured and multiply if they find an organic substance they feed on or a damp, dark corner. They are tiny, airborne and cause allergy. Pets can also be a source of allergen. Tiny hairs of pets were believed to be a cause of allergy. Dr. John Ohman of Boston proved that these animals lick themselves, and dried saliva coated on their hair is airborne. When they fly and are inhaled by or come in contact with allergy sufferers asthma results. Cats which lick themselves by the hour are a bigger source of allergens than dogs. The most common and important airborne allergens present outside the house is pollen. "Anemophilous Plants" are those plants which disperse their pollen by wind, have their flowers and anthers arranged and modified in such a way that the pollen are non-sticky and their size very small, so that they are easily dispersed in air. Ten Thousand pollen of the 'forget-me-not' plant could together make a pinhead. They can be carried very high due to the buoyancy in the air and can travel many miles. Grasses like *Bermuda*, and *Imperata*; weeds like palthenium, amaranthus, xanthium, artemisia, chenopodium; trees like cassia siamea, albinzia, holoptelia and castor are most common plants whose pollen are easily airborne and cause allergy.

Allergies and Dogs

People with allergies can tolerate certain breeds of dogs, particularly poodles, airedale, terriers, portuguese water dogs and terriers which do not shed hairs. Dog dandex or flakes of skin cause allergy (not hair of dogs). They say dandex sticks to hair and with less hair being shed, less dandex is in air. A type of toy spaniel called Bichon Frise looks like a poodle and is allergy proof. Bichons do not shed dandex and are very compatible to allergic members in family. In sensitive people sometimes allergies develop at any time even after a long time exposure to an animal. Chihuahua theory is very prevalent. Classic folklore tale in America is that Chihuahuas actually cure asthma. This safe pet theory is wrong. They are sort of dreadful little dogs. They wheeze when they breathe and people assume dogs were drawing evil spirits out of asthma patients and taking it into themselves. Actually safe breed theories are wishful thinking. Proteins in animal skin secretions and saliva make people allergic to dogs or cats. There is *no exception*, say doctors.

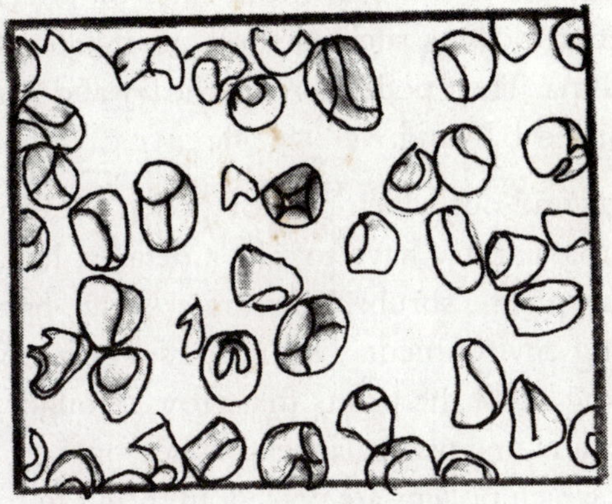

Fig. 3.1 : Magnified Pollen Grains of a Grass (major cause of hay fever)

Extrinsic Asthma

Extrinsic asthma, atopic asthma or the allergic asthma occurs due to allergy to various substances. In this chapter, we will be discussing about the allergic asthma in detail. One of the most important points to be recalled here is that the substances causing allergic asthma do not fall into any one category. They can be diverse and come from different classes of substances.

Plant Pollens

Pollen grains are yellow granules seen in some flowers. Only some of the pollens cause asthma. All the pollens do not cause allergy. Only some pollens bring out the allergic manifestations. For a pollen of a plant to cause an allergy, it must be carried by the wind for pollination purposes. For this reason, it must be very light in weight; also the pollens must be produced in abundance. Pollens are released from the flowers very early in the morning, often before the sunrise. Hence many patients of asthma, sensitive to pollens, have their symptoms in the early morning. Different asthma patients are allergic to different pollens. Most of the patients are allergic to more than one kind of pollen. Pollens of common garden flowers such as roses, marigold, phlox, etc. do not cause asthma. Their pollens are too heavy and large and hence cannot be carried by wind.

In order to find out which type of pollen is causing allergy in an asthmatic patient, we have to take a detailed history of which are the various plants, shrubs, trees grasses, etc., present near his house/working environment. This needs surveying, identification and cataloguing of all the plants that grow through- out the year (annual) or in any one particular season (seasonal). Then we have to determine which pollens are present in the air in the area under study in different months of the year using 'Pollen Catchers' (glass slides coated with vaseline are placed on this specialised instrument called Pollen Catcher). Pollen catchers are placed on strategic locations where there is free flow of air. Pollens in the air get stuck to the vaseline on the slides. The slides are examined under a microscope and the type and nature of pollens, their number, etc., are evaluated. This study gives data regarding :

1) Type of pollens present (qualitative data).
2) Their number (quantitative data).
3) The month they are present (Pollen Calendar).

This kind of pollen studies are done daily, throughout the year, and for about five years on stretch. Pollen calendar is very important for investigations of asthma. A patient presenting with symptoms of allergic asthma in the months of March (spring time) may be allergic to some pollens present in air at that time. From the qualitative data, we can know which is the culprit plant, flower or weed.

Some studies done in Delhi show that pollens are abundant in air in autumn, spring, early summer, i.e., from April to September. Less pollens are found in air from June to August. Asthma patients feel exacerbations (during high pollen in air months) and remissions (during the low pollen in air months). In Delhi studies, trees like *Salvadoha*, *Terminalia*, *Ricinus* have been contributing to a lot of pollens in air. Weeds like xanthium, cannabis and amaranthus also contribute significantly. Grasses like *Eynoden sorghum* also bring out a sizable number of pollens into the air. Rainfall, temperature, sunshine, wind speed, wind direction also increase or decrease pollen population in a particular area. Rainfall has a double effect on pollens. During the pollen season they wash away the pollens and its quantity in air. On the other hand, if rainfall is heavy before pollination, they stimulate profuse growth of plants and pollen production.

People are rarely allergic to large heavy pollen grains of flowers which are not carried by wind but by insects.

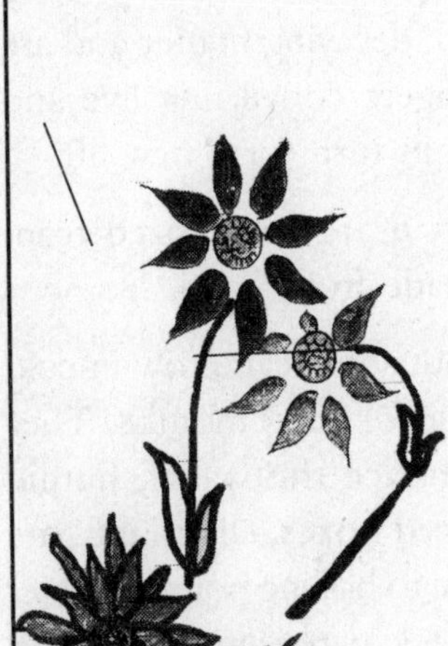

- The most common allergens are actually the pollens in spring and grass pollens in summer and ray weed pollens in fall.
- Some pollen seasons are worse than the others. Summers that follow long wet springs can be unbearable to people with grass allergies.
- Pollens counts often included in local weather report tends to be high on warm dry days and low on wet cool days.
- Mild winters in normally cold climates make for a bumper crop of tree pollen in string.
- When pollen counts soar even people who are not allergic strongly may develop a reaction.

* One should avoid going outside during early morning when the pollen count is at its highest. If one does go out, he can wear a dust mask to avoid pollen allergy.

Pollen on Your Plate?

If you have hay fever, certain foods may worsen your allergy attacks or trigger an itchy tongue, mouth or throat. The following foods contain proteins similar to those in certain pollens. Keep a food diary to determine if they affect you.

Pollen Trigger	*Foods to Avoid*
Ragweed	Contaloupes, bananas, cucumbers, watermelons, honeydew melons
Grass	Apples, carrots, celery, oranges, tomatoes, watermelons
Birch tree	Apples, carrots, celery, cherries, fennel, hazelnuts, oranges, pears, potatoes, walnuts, Maple syrup.

Fungi

Fungi are simple plants, small in size. They have no green pigment (chlorophyll), hence they cannot make their own food. Fungi have a slender branch like growing vegetative part called mycelia. They reproduce by spores. They feed on dead, decaying matter and are called Saprophytes. They act as scavengers converting live and dead matter into basic chemicals which in turn form new life.

Antibiotics like penicillin, streptomycin are synthesized from fungi. Alcohol, wine, cheese etc., are made from fungi.

Fungi grow between 20° and 32°C, but some can grow in cold temperatures. They can survive freezing for long months. They need 70 per cent humidity to grow, hence the warm, humid conditions in rooms, storage places, closed boxes, shoes, etc., are ideal for their growth. Temperatures close to boiling point of water can easily kill most of them. Fungi attack paper, wood, etc. In homes furniture dust, mattress dust are good harbourers of fungi. Home gardens breed fungal spores constantly. They grow abundantly on rotting leaves, foliage areas. Where grains are grown or stored also have an immense number of fungal spores. In India, cow and buffalo dung (*gobar*) are still used as domestic fuel and these form one of the principal source materials of fungi. Foods such as cheese use fungi for their distinctive taste. Beer, wine, bread, cakes, etc., are all manufactured using yeast, but fungi can enter food as contaminants also. Baked foods often become mouldy in humid weather. Potatoes, onions also are common sources of fungal contamination. Fungal spores are very light in weight and are carried and disseminated by the wind. All the viable fungal spores in the air are not allergenic. Important allergenic fungi are:

1) *Aspergillus tamarii*

2) *Aspergillus fumigatus*

3) *Candida*

4) *Mucor and phoma.*

Mould

The ugly, furry stuff that grows in damp spots around your house can be either mould or mildew. These pernicious plant fungi damage walls, shoes, fabrics, and shed microscopic spores into the air that irritate the people who are allergic to them. When inhaled by a sensitive person, some mildew/mould spores can trigger allergic reactions such as congestion, itchy eyes, watery eyes, breathing difficulty. In very rare cases, exposure may cause Hypersensitivity Pneunonitis which can lead to serious heart and lung problems or a dangerous condition in infants known as Pulmonary Hemosiderosis or bleeding lung syndrome.

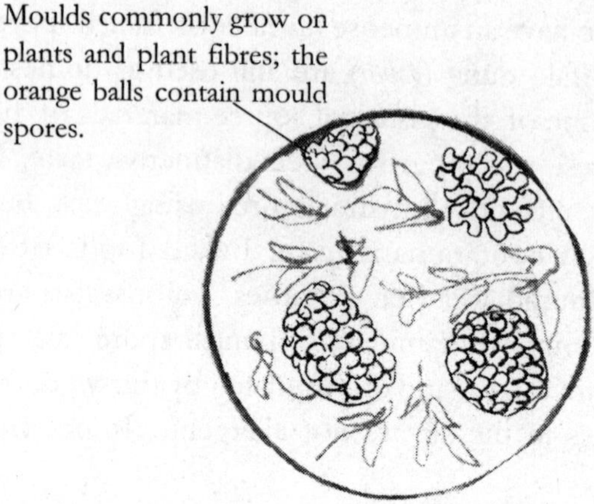

Clean up mould with hydrogen peroxide, white vinegar,etc. Weara protective mask and rubber gloves. Discard mouldy breadsrefrigerated foods. Moulds can leach unseen toxins into food.

Fungal spores present in air rank second (first being the pollens) in causing allergy-induced asthma. A doctor treating the fungus sensitive patients must have knowledge of various fungi, their concentration, seasons when they are present. Like a pollen calendar, a fungal calendar can be constructed and followed. Surveys in Delhi show that fungal spore concentration is very high during November and April (during autumn and spring). In rainy season, fungal concentration goes down as rain washes away the spores. Cladosporium spores have been found in large numbers in slides prepared in Delhi.

A fungus-sensitive patient shows certain common features. He has symptoms throughout the year. Symptoms increase during the increase in concentration of spores. (For example, in Delhi, it may be in November and April). They can be diagnosed as having fungus spore-induced asthma by eliminating other allergens from their history. Suppose they are not allergic to pollens, house dust, then fungal spores can be a possible candidate. Persons developing symptoms on exposure to compost, dead leaves and foliage, hay, while harvesting or ploughing are surely the ones allergic to spores. Some patients give a history of consuming mould-containing foods prior to developing symptoms. This is self-explanatory and it is easy to diagnose.

Mould-sensitive patients may sometimes be also allergic to other allergens like pollens, house dust, etc. Such patients who develop bronchial asthma on exposure to fungal spores, must avoid basements, humid, warm areas. They should see to it that all rooms inside the house are well ventilated and that the walls of the household do not absorb moisture. Painted walls are preferred. Walls can be plastered too. Potted plants should not be kept inside the house as the soils of potted house plants and the plants itself become infected with fungi.

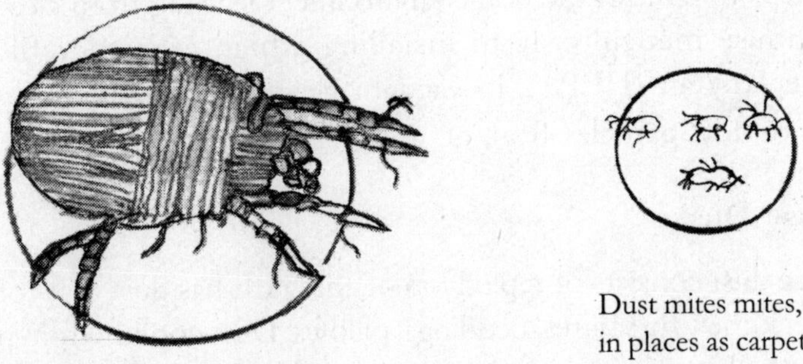

(Magnified about 600 times)

Dust mites mites, live in places as carpeting, mattresses and pillows

Fig. 3.2 : Dustmite

House dust typically contains minute particles of human skin, hair, saliva; animal hair and dander; insect parts and faeces; and fibres from upholstery, carpets and clothing. The mixture plays hast to moulds, viruses and bacteria, but the worst health threat for many people come from microscopic insects called dustmites or more specifically from their droppings. These mites (a single pinch of dust contain thousands) feed on the skin flakes shed by humans. Found even in spotless homes, they are especially dangerous for asthma sufferers because breathing in their droppings can trigger attacks and contribute to the development of diseases.

Allergic reactions to dust occur commonly in both adults and children. All the allergic symptoms, like wheezing, sneezing, runny nose, water eyes, fatigue, cough, itchy rash can occur.

Symptoms occur alone or in combination often making the allergy difficult to identify. Only a doctor can arrive at the correct diagnosis.

House dust breeds a broad spectrum of harmful micro-organisms. In Canada, this is a big problem. Since the Canadians spend up to 90 per cent of their day indoors (according to a survey), these contaminants create significant health risks by harbouring bacteria-causing allergic reactions and aggravating those who suffer from asthma.

Steps to control the home environment starting from cleaning the house meticulously to installing a high efficiency filters, particularly air (HEPA), in vacuum cleaner, air purifier etc., to remove dust particles from air are followed.

House Dust

House dust consists of a plethora of things. It has dust that comes from clothes, furnitures, beddings, pillows. Dust coming from pets, from the fungi spores can be seen on house dust. Insects killed or damaged can be seen as small remnants in the house dust. Human skin, hair are also seen in house dust. Outside dust, via wind, also enters house dust. Old furnitures, carpets, rugs contribute a great deal of house dust. Seen in the shafts of sunlight entering a room (tyndall effect), these particles settle down in the form of house dust.

In 1964, a Dutch research team demonstrated that it was the common house dust mite called Dermotopagoides Pteronyssinus that was causing 'allergy' in house dust. Later other allergenic mites were discovered in the house. Samples of house dust have shown up to 200 mites in 1 gm of it.

Mites feed and grow on contents of house dust. The common house mite is very small. It grows well in high humidities and at an optimal temperature of 25°C. It can become airborne during the cleaning of the house, making of bed. Some asthmatic patients improve on admission to hospital. This is probably due to removal from the house dust environment. Some persons show an aggravation of their symptoms in bed or bedroom. This is associated with house dust and house mite concentration being more in the bed and bedroom. Persons allergic to house dust can be allergic to pollens, fungal spores, etc. also. Patients allergic to house dust :

1) must avoid dusty areas; bedroom must be very clean;
2) must remove all rugs, carpets, curtains, dust catching objects or these objects must be vacuum cleaned daily;
3) must have the room cleaned with a wet cloth;
4) must have clean closets containing clothes and must have minimum things;
5) must have pillows made of foam rubber.

Food Articles

Food allergy is a well documented phenomenon. Hippocrates, 'The father of medicine', the famous Greek physician, was the first to record a case of stomach upset and skin allergy in a patient who had consumed milk. The Greek physician Galen too described a case of allergy to goat's milk. All these were in ancient times and this proves the ancient nature of these food allergies.

The patient can produce a variety of symptoms on consuming a food to which he is sensitive. This can be itching, sores in mouth, vomiting, diarrhoea, headache, etc. Symptoms around the mouth may appear without delay while the other symptoms appear much later. Other allergic factors can also add to the effects of food. Some food produce allergic symptoms immediately and in some cases allergic symptoms appear only late. Food allergy is more common in infants and children. Adults who are allergic to food are found to have additional allergy to pollens, house dust, fungal spores, etc.

Milk, egg, wheat and fish are the common food products which produce allergy in sensitive individuals. Cow's milk is not an uncommon allergen in infancy as it is the major foreign protien food in the early months of life. Milk allergy according to a statistical figure occurs in 0.5 per cent of children. Milk allergy manifests as a 'feeling of being unwell' in most of the infants. Other manifestations are symptoms of GIT and respiratory tract. Eczema and urticaria can be the other symptoms. Mother's milk is the best treatment for this. Till the age of nine months to a year cow's milk is best avoided. The diagnosis of milk allergy can be established in a baby by stopping the milk from diet; note for 'complete absence of symptoms'. Then rechallenge the baby with milk. Note for "coming back of symptoms". This hide and seek technique clinches the diagnosis of milk allergy. Once the diagnosis is established the offending milk is removed from the diet. Soyabean milk is the best substitute. After the baby becomes a year old a trial with cow's milk can be done. If the child does not tolerate it once again soyabean milk is given. If a baby tolerates cow's milk with few symptoms cow's milk can be given in slowly increasing graded quantities.

Wheat allergy manifests as rashes, abdominal colic, diarrhoea. Eczema and asthmatic attacks can occur in older children. Wheat is given as cereal, so this can be substituted with some other cereal. It can be re-introduced and seen for symptoms. The white of an egg is a protein called albumin. This being a foreign protein can cause reactions if a person is allergic to it. Raw egg consumption can cause even shock, fainting and collapse in sensitive individuals. Nuts like almonds, walnuts, cashewnuts, etc., can also produce allergy. Fruits like apples, bananas, oranges, lemons, grapes; vegetables like onions, radish, mushrooms; jaggery, mustard, chocolates, watermelons, cucumber, soft drinks are some of the other foods people are found allergic to.

Diagnosis is done by (1) detail history (2) eliminating the diet and looking for symptoms (3) studying a patient's food habits and studying the symptoms associated with it. The patient must know the ingredients of the food he consumes and must avoid it in any form. For example, a person allergic to eggs must avoid cakes, cookies, etc., having egg.

Treatment includes avoiding the food which is causing allergy in the individual. He can take a substitute (for example, soyabean milk for cow's milk, cane sugar for jaggery). Cooked foods are prescribed as the raw foods are more allergenic whereas cooked (hence denatured) foods are less allergenic.

Insects

Insect Bite Allergy (IBA) is not very uncommon. Insect bites produce pain, swelling and also allergic reactions due to the 'Antigenic' nature of venom in some individuals. Insects are classified as stinging and biting insects.

Mosquitoes, sandfly, etc., are biting insects. They produce a delayed allergic reaction. They cause redness, swelling at the bitten site several hours later. Reactions are not very serious. Antihistamines can be given to decrease itching. No further treatment is needed, whereas bee, wasps are stinging insects and produce immediate allergic reactions. Symptoms can vary from local redness, swelling at the site of stinging to generalised swelling, urticaria, choking, fainting and even fatal consequences. The best approach is 'prevention is better than cure.' Avoiding places/situations where one can be stung by insects; keeping the body covered while going outdoors; if stung careful removal of sting from the site using a needle is advised. If the sting is on a limb, tying a tight bandage to compress blood vessels and prevent spread of venom in body is done. Care should be taken to tie the bandage tightly just *above the site of the sting*. This tourniquet should be loosened every five minutes and can be removed after half an hour. Icepacks and antihistamine tablets are other treatments. Adrenaline is recommended only in severe reactions to stings. Hyposensitisation against sting venoms is nowadays done and has given very good results. Bits and pieces of small dead insects in dust can also be a source of allergy. These remnants of insects can ever trigger an asthmatic attack in allergic individuals. During monsoon, millions of insects appear for a day and die. These disintegrated insects become part of dust, like a pollen. Fungus calendar an insect calendar can also be made (for the particular season what are the insects seen, their breeding period, lifespan, etc.) and a person's symptoms can be correlated with these calendars to determine the culprit.

Symptoms of a bee sting include hives, breathing difficulties, light-headedness, swelling of the tongue or on the throat, nausea, severe headache. This calls for emergency medical help. A delay in treatment could be fatal.

People who suspect they are allergic to a bee sting should go to a doctor and get a skin test done. If the test is +ve, desensitisation may be recommended. Wearing a medic alert bracelet and carrying a ready-to-inject syringe of epinephrine (available by prescription) are recommended. If a person is stung, he can inject this medication. This will give him time to rush to an emergency room for observation and treatment (Rx).

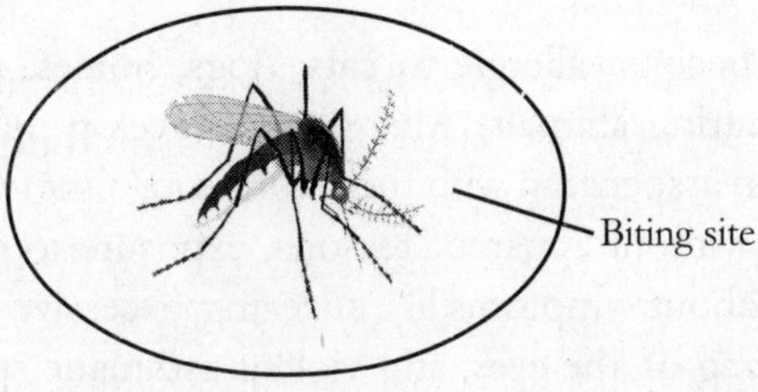

Fig. 3.4 : Biting Insect (Mosquito)

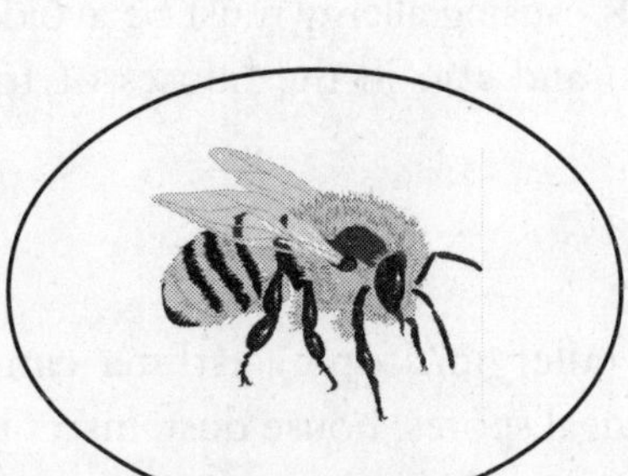

Fig. 3.5 : Stinging Insect (Bee)

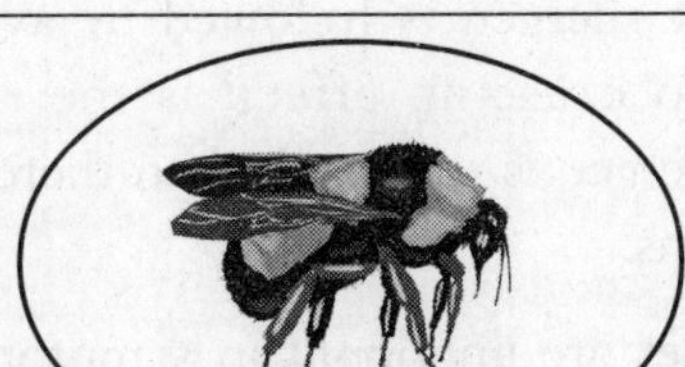

More than 100 North Americans die of bee

Allergic to Bee Strings ?

About 15 per cent of North Americans are potentially allergic to bee venom. For many of them a sting will result in greater than usual pain and itching. But for more people with severe allergies bee stings can trigger a life-threatening condition, i.e., *anaphylactic shock*.

Animals

One can become allergic to cats, dogs, horses, fur-bearing and feather-bearing animals. Allergy can develop in a person (who has been in association with them for a long time) to these animals. Suddenly without apparent reasons, exposure to animal allergens can bring about symptoms like sneezing, excessive itching, burning and watering of the eyes, and violent asthmatic spasms. Removal of the cause (here the particular animal) is the main line of treatment. Some persons are allergic both to dust in house and animals. In such cases, the cause being double symptoms will be very severe. Animals causing allergy must be avoided in the house (if it is pet animals) and also in the houses of friends, relatives, neighbours.

Summary

i) Extrinsic (allergic/atopic) asthma can be caused by pollens, fungal spores, house dust, insect bites and stings, food substances, animals, etc.

ii) Detection of the causative 'allergen' is very important. A person allergic to two or more allergens has to be carefully evaluated.

iii) Detection of allergen is followed by avoidance of the allergen. 'No cause-no effect' is the rule. So, if the offending allergen is removed, then there are no allergic manifestations.

iv) Antihistamines are important in symptomatic treatment of many allergies. Hyposensitisation too is beneficial.

v) 'Prevent rather than cure' is the rule. Avoid the cause rather than getting treated after suffering.

4

EXTRINSIC ASTHMA : CONTRIBUTORY FACTORS

Facts on Asthma

1) One statistics says that children with one asthmatic parent contract asthma at three to six times the rate of other kids. Those with two asthmatic parents have 10 times the risk, and identical twins are more likely than fraternal twins to share allergies.

2) The prevalence of asthma has doubled in India in the last 190 yrs. It is expected to tripple in the next five to 10 years.

Factors Influencing Asthma

Bronchial asthma, which has become a fairly common condition, is influenced by many factors. Estimates put the figure as roughly 1 per cent of the world's population. That is the number of people affected by bronchial asthma. It affects both sexes equally and is more prevalent in the upper strata or higher income group of the society. In this chapter, we will be discussing some of the factors which influence bronchial asthma.

Heredity

Asthma occurs in a person with a family history of disease. The greater the degree of inheritance, the greater the chances for the offsprings to become sensitive. If both the father and mother are affected, the disease surfaces in the children even before they attain puberty. Allergic predisposition is inherited and not the particular allergic disease itself. Suppose the parent has hay fever, the children need not necessarily develop hay fever, but may get eczema due to the inheritance of allergic characteristics.

Infection

ACTIVE INFECTION
↓
Exacerbates an asthmatic condition

Mechanism I

Subsided infection
↓
Symptoms of asthma also subsides

Mechanism II

Infection
↓
Activates sensitivity to a specific allergen
↓
Manifestation of allergy even after infection subsides

The above charts show two mechanisms. In mechanism 1, an infection, when active, brings out or exacerbates an asthmatic attack. A child may become breathless, develop wheezing, etc., but once the infection subsides, symptoms of asthma also subsides. In mechanism 2 due to activation of sensitivity or allergy mechanisms, there is an asthmatic attack continuing even after the infection subsides.

Excessive mucous and other secretions (in patients of allergic rhinitis, asthma) in lungs, nose favours growth of micro-organisms and make these patients predisposed to chest infections. Allergy and infection set up a vicious cycle and one aggravates the other. Infections aggravate asthma. Asthma favouring growth of micro-organisms can end up as an emphysema or chronic bronchitis. Both need treatment. Infection should be treated with antibiotics and allergy with anti-allergic measures.

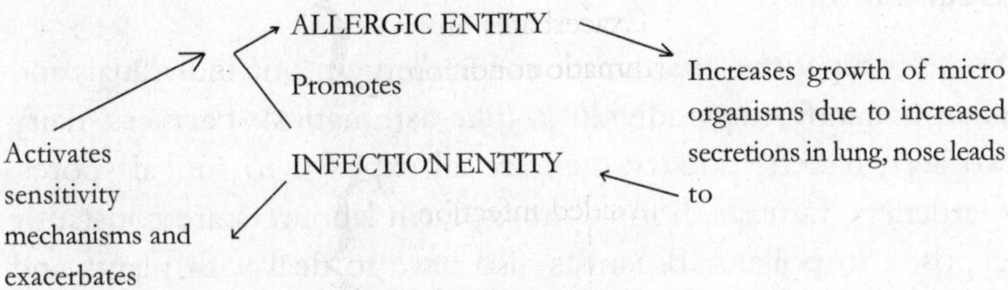

Fig. 4.1 : Vicious Cycle

Emotional States

Any excessive emotional reaction precipitates an attack of asthma in a person predisposed to it. A traumatic event can trigger an asthmatic attack and even after the event is long over, its memories can bring out a fresh attack. Conversely, a person in a traumatic emotional set-up, getting asthmatic attacks, once removed from that set-up and put in a calm environment sometimes shows improvement. Probably the no-cause-no-effect theory can be applied here.

Climate

Dry climate is better for an asthmatic than a humid one. Rainy weather can have a double impact. For some asthmatics increased humidity during the rainy weather exacerbates their symptoms, but for those asthmatics who are allergic to pollen, rain brings remission as it washes down all the pollen. Asthmatics feel better away from a seacoast.

Early mornings aggravate symptoms in asthmatics as this is the time when flowers open and discharge their pollens. Winds from particular directions may be carrying pollens sensitive to patients and this may precipitate an attack. Fall in barometric pressure (as before a thunderstorm) is not suitable for asthmatics. Altitudes also influence asthmatic attacks. When an asthmatic patient goes up a hill, his symptoms improve because of a changed environment, changes in flora/pollens and lessened dust.

Occupation

Some occupations are hazardous for allergy-prone individuals and allergy-manifesting individuals (like asthmatics). Farmers, dairy workers, bakers, poultry men are all exposed to fungal spores. Gardeners, farmers, horticulturists, farm labourers are constantly exposed to pollens. Botanists also have to deal with plants and flowers. Upholsterers, mattress renovaters, painters, carpenters are exposed to large quantities of house dust. Flour mill workers are exposed to dust with various kinds of particles in it. Barbers, beauty parlour maids are exposed to animal dander.

For a patient who has asthma, such occupations can exacerbate his symptoms. A person who has allergic background on exposure to such substances as pollens, dust, spores due to a particular occupation will see that his symptoms of allergy are being brought out/manifested.

An offending agent does not precipitate asthma on the first exposure. A sensitisation period ranging from a few months to years ensues, during which antibodies develop. On the second exposure, the attack manifests, like active and passive smoking. Certain occupations cause allergy symptoms and manifestations not only in active workers, but also in people who live in the neighbourhood. This becomes a public health problem. A factory manufacturing a particular product may cause allergic symptoms for people living around it. A person who is an asthmatic should choose a proper profession and also a proper neighbourhood to live, as both these are important contributory factors to increasing or decreasing intensity of his condition.

Allergy prone individual

↘ on exposure to

Hazardous occupation

↙ becomes

Allergy-manifested individual

↘

Exposed to hazardous occupation

↘

Symptoms exacerbated.

Glandular disturbances which accompany pregnancy, menstruation and menopause can also contribute to the severity of an asthmatic attack.

Summary

1) Factors contributing to asthma are many.
2) Heredity, allergic trait, is inherited, not the disease proper.
3) Infection and allergy form a vicious cycle.
4) Emotions exacerbate a attack; a calm set-up decreases symptoms.
5) Climate, rain, humidity, pressure, wind all are important factors affecting an asthmatic patient's health.
6) Occupations aggravating or precipitating an allergic attack have to be avoided; 'living place' to be selected keeping the neighbourhood in mind.
7) Pregnancy, menopause-associated glandular problems affect an attack of asthma.

5

EXTRINSIC ASTHMA : DIAGNOSIS AND TREATMENT

Diagnosis and Treatment of Asthma

First and foremost comes a detailed history of the patient. Breathlessness is to be evaluated for asthma.

Allergy	→	to what he is allergic to	
	→	in which season symptoms	exacerbate / undergo remission
	→	symptoms to be correlated with allergens being discussed	
Symptoms	→	what are they, when they started, what triggers them, what precipitates them, etc.	

After the above points are noted down, lab tests are the next in the list. These lab tests and case history help in finding the allergenic factors.

Skin Tests

These are done to detect the presence of antibodies (reagins). These antibodies are located in blood and skin. In skin tests antigen (allergen) is applied on the skin. If there is a specific antibody for this antigen, there is an antigen-antibody union (Ag-Ab complex).

This releases chemicals like histamine from the tissues and results in a weal and redness around the test site.

Skin Test

Antigen (allergen)

↓

applied to the skin which may or not have antibodies (reagin) to the specific antigen applied

↙ ↘

If Ab is present then Ag-Ab complex is formed	If Ab is absent no Ag-Ab complex
↓	↓
Release of histamine and other chemicals from tissues	No release
↓	↓
Weal and redness around test site	No weal/no redness
↓	↓
Skin test positive	Skin test negative

Skin tests are done with dusts, pollens, moulds. Extracts of these common allergens are prepared and used. The extracts used must be (1) active and potent (2) free from micro-organisms (3) should have only a negligeble amount of any irritant. The crude antigens are reduced to a fine powder, treated with acetone to remove fats and then is treated with with a watery solvent. The resultant product is dialised. Concentration, neutralisation, standardisation follow and the extract with natural antigen characteristics is ready for use. Skin tests are done by scratch or intracutaneous methods. In a scratch test, small scratches are made on the forearm and allergenic extracts are applied on these scratches. After 15 to 20 minutes, these are removed and test sites are observed and evaluated. Control tests with 'allergenic principle devoid diluents' are there for comparison. An important point to remember is that the scratch mode should only be superficial. In the intracutaneous method, sterile allergenic extracts in quantity of 0.02ml are introduced into the skin by a syringe. Reactions are more prominent in this method and it is a children-safe painless technique.

The skin test reactions are graded from 0, 1, 2, 3 to 4 plus depending upon the degree of swelling and redness produced. A positive reaction of significance must correlate with the clinical history, symptoms and other findings of the/in the patient.

Table 5.1 : Grading of Skin Test

Grade	*Size of Weal*	*Size of Redness*
0	Same as control	Same as control
1+	2 times more than control	10-20 mm
2+	3 times more than control	20-30 mm
3+	4 times more than control	more than 30 mm
4+	5 times more than control	more than 40 mm

Negative reactions indicate absence of antibody against allergen tested; but use of inadequate or weak extract can also give false negative results.

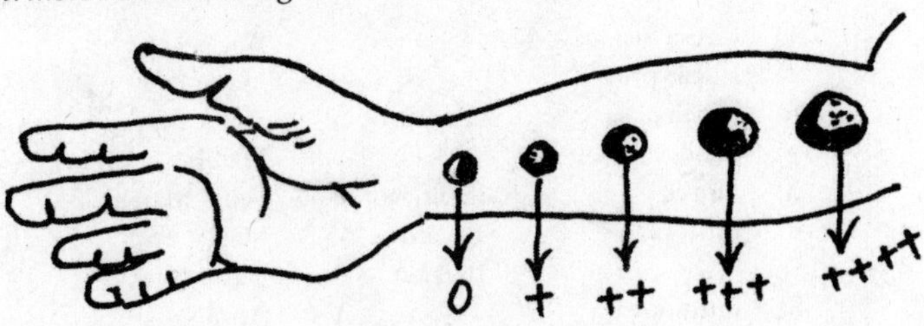

Fig. 5.1 : Grading of Skin Tests

Table 5.2 : Skin Testing Chart

Name of the patient :________________ Date : __________

		Allergens: English name	*Local Name*	*Months in which present in Delhi air*	*Grading 0, 1+, 2+ 3+, 4+*
I Pollens					
Grasses:	1)	Cenchrus	Aujan	July - Oct.	
	2)	Cynoden	Doob	Year around	
	3)	Pennisetum	Bajra	Aug. - Sept.	
	4)	Sorghum	Jawar	Aug. - Sept.	
Weeds:	1)	Adhatoda	Rusa	Dec. - Jan.	
	2)	Ageratum	Neelum	Dec. - Apr.	
	3)	Amaranthus Spinosus	Kately Chauli	Year around	
	4)	Argemone	Peeli Kateli	Jan. - March	
	5)	Artemisia	—	Sept. - Oct.	
	6)	Asphodelus	Piazi	Jan. - March	
	7)	Brassica	Sarson	Dec. - March	
	8)	Cannabis Indica	Bhang	July - Sept.	
	9)	Chenopodium Album	Bathuva	Dec. - March	
	10)	Dodonea Mehendi	Vilaiti	Jan. - Feb.	
	11)	Parthenium	—	Year around	
	12)	Xanthium	Choota Gokhru	Sept. - April	

(Contd ...)

Trees:	1)	Cassia Siamea	—	Aug. - Feb.
	2)	Eucalyptus	Safeda	May - Feb.
	3)	Kigelia	Zarphanoos	Apr. - May
	4)	Melia	Bakain	March
	5)	Morus	Shahtoot	Feb. - March
	6)	Prosopis	Vilaiti	Mar. - April
			Kikkar	Sep. - Nov.
	7)	Putranjiva	—	April
	8)	Ricinus	Arandi	Year around
	9)	Salvadora	Peelu	Nov. - March.
II Dust	1)	House Dust	—	
	2)	Paper Dust	—	
	3)	Wheat Dust	—	
	4)	Cotton Dust	—	
III Fungi	1)	Alternaria	—	Year around
	2)	Aspergillus Fumigatus		Sept. - Nov.
	3)	Candida	—	May - Nov.
	4)	Cladosporium	—	Sept. - Nov.
	5)	Helminthosporium	—	Feb. - June
	6)	Mucor	—	May - Oct.
	7)	Phoma	—	Oct. - Nov.

Pollen Watch

Bangalore (Karnataka) has a high incidence of allergic pathologies. The weather is an important factor. It being the garden city, there is a lot of Avenue trees, flowers which supply the source of allergy. Aerobiology and allergy lab, botany department in Bangalore University monitors the pollen in Bangalore atmosphere. The pollen watch statistics is published in the paper every week for informing the people and 'creating awareness' among them.

POLLEN WATCH

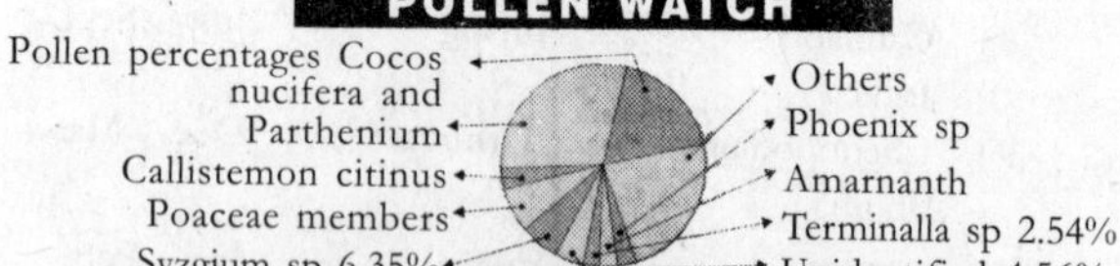

MOULD WATCH

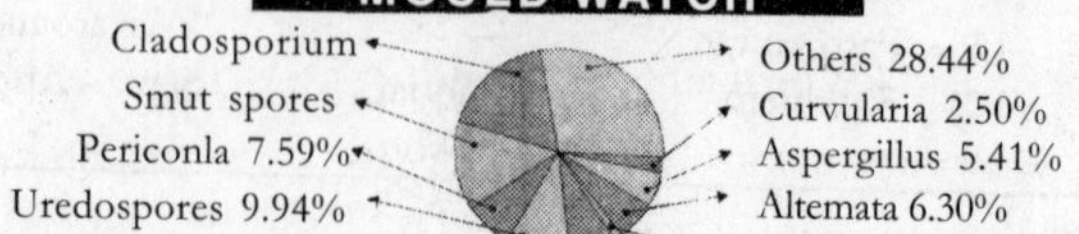
Cladosporium
Smut spores
Periconla 7.59%
Uredospores 9.94%
Nigmspora 7.15%
Others 28.44%
Curvularia 2.50%
Aspergillus 5.41%
Altemata 6.30%
Unidentified 1.30%

> This week's pollen monitoring of Bangalore atmosphere by using Rotorod intermitten volumetric sampler operated at the Meterological Centre on Palace Road, indicates a considerable increase in the total pollen count to 236, equivalent to the density of 72.75 per cub metre of air sampled. Pollen of Congress weed, Parthenium hysterophorus (30.11%), has bounced back to the first position followed by pollen of *Cocos nucifera* (18.22%) and other palms.
>
> Many Fabaceae (formerly Leguminosae) members are in full bloom now. This is reflected by fairly high pollen count of *Caesalpinia sp.* (8.48%), *Mimosa pudica* (7.62%). Pollen of *Callistemon citrinus* (bottlebrush plant) makes significant appearance by contributing 3.38 per cent of pollen population. Grass pollen (Poaceae members) have been represented only by 7.20 per cent.
>
> Bangalore has been experiencing fairly warm and windy weather. This may be the reason for higher pollen and mould spore count. Total mould spore count has gone up to 4,432, equivalent to density of 1,368.1 per cubic metre of air sampled. This ratio of pollen and mould spores this week is 1:18. Cladosporium (17.49%), Smut spores (13.88%), Periconia (7.59%) and Alternaria (6.30%) lead the mould spore count. There is a slight increase in Uredospores count at 9.94 per cent.
>
> Spores of Powdery mildew make significant appearance (9.36%) this week.
>
> A clipping of one such 'pollen watch' has been given earlier. This was for the month of January 2001, dated 24th. The data gives us the names of various flora, weed, etc. It has also given us data on 'mould spores count' as fungal spores are also carried by wind. These kind of pollen/mould spore monitoring is very helpful in diagnosis, treatment and prevention of allergic disorders.

After detailed history skin tests comes the Provocation Inhalation Tests. In order to confirm doubts in positive skin reaction, some doctors perform Provocative Inhalation Tests. The extract which gave a doubtful positive test is given to the patient for inhalation. Whether the patient gets breathless after inhaling it or not is noted. The spasm of airways produced as a result of positive reaction is measured by making the patient take a breath test called 'Spirometry'.

This test along with the skin test information gives valuable data about the culprit allergen, but this test is not safe and can turn 'Iatrogenic' (when a test procedure itself induces a pathology) inducing a severe attack of asthma in some patients. This test is always done in a well-equipped hospital which can handle respiratory emergencies.

Before going into the discussion of treatment, we must follow the proverb "Self help is the best help" and "God helps those who Help Themselves". We will briefly discuss how a person can answer a question whether he is a potential asthmatic or not. The following chart is a 'Self Help' chart for a person to assess his status regarding his potential to develop asthma.

ARE YOU A POTENTIAL ASTHMATIC?

(Answer Yes/No)

1) Is there a history of asthma in your family ?
2) Do you have throat or nose infections very often ?
3) Do you get bouts of sneezing at the change of season ?
4) Do you experience breathing difficulty when exposed to a cold-wind-swept environment ?
5) Do you have a running nose constantly ?
6) Does the change of season cause coughing and throat irritation ?
7) Do you get skin rash and itching very often for reasons known or unknown ?
8) Do you live or work in a pollution-ridden environment ?
9) Do you experience a choking feeling when you are tensed or depressed ?
10) Does even mild exertion give you breathlessness ?

The more 'Yes' answers one gives, the more prone one is to the disease.

Once a person has gone through the above chart and before he wants further information on asthma, he would like to have some idea on various signs and symptoms of the disease. Asthma in your children is not always easy for parents to identify (or even for doctors to diagnose) since sometimes it can masquerade as a cold or respiratory infection. Some possible red flags are:

1) Wheezing

This seems like an obvious tip off but two-thirds of infants under one year old who wheeze with respiratory infections do not become asthmatic. If wheezing recurs constantly, however, it may be asthma.

2) Serious Coughs

Coughing is an *inescapable part* of life, but persistent hacking, particularly accompanied by wheezing, is a clear warning. Croup can be another signal if the child has it more than once. Among the common causes of asthma in children are (as discussed earlier) food, whereas these are responsible for only a small per cent of cases among adults.

3) Play-related Problems

If exercise or playing hard typically brings on a fit of coughing, tightness in the chest or more than the usual panting, asthma mat be to blame.

4) Trouble Breathing at Night

It is not only bad dreams that spook asthmatic kids. If shortness of breath awakens them at night, suspect asthma.

5) Family History

We have already discussed this. If one parent has asthma, the child is at least three times more likely to have inherited the disease. A strong family history of hay fever and eczema may be another tip off.

Some Do's and Don'ts for asthmatics:

Do's

1) Keep the environment, particularly the bedroom, dust- free.
2) Replace dust-collecting furnishing carpets, curtains, bedcovers, with easy-to-wash synthetic material.
3) Use blankets made of synthetic fibre.
4) Sleep in a room that is airy and has proper ventilation.
5) Take light meals before going to bed at night. A full stomach makes breathing difficult.

6) Drink frequently warm water or other beverages that go well with you.
7) Follow regular daily routine meals, working hours, and going to bed.
8) Avoid tension-generating situations that can trigger an asthma attack.

Don'ts

1) Go outdoor during a pollen boom and pollen prolific months.
2) Stay in or near a humid environment which is laced with asthma-aggravating and asthma-triggering fungi.
3) Expose yourself to known and identified allergens.
4) Consume foods that are known to produce allergenic reactions—fish, eggs, nuts, food preservatives.
5) Go for a walk in areas swept by cold winds.
6) Play with pet dogs, cats, etc., which produce allergic reactions.
7) Ignore throat irritations, nasal blokades and delay medical help.
8) Smoke cigarettes, cigars, etc.
9) Take alcoholic beverages as far as possible.

Drug Treatment of Asthma : A Quick Review

Sympathoninetics

Drugs which are for treatment of bronchial asthma in this group are salbutamol, salmeterol, adrenaline, ephedrine, terbutaline, orciprenaline, isoprenaline. These drugs do not provide immediate relief of bronchospasm because their onset of action is slow. They are used in maintenance therapy. These drugs produce bronchodilatation by acting on β_2 adrenergic receptors present in bronchial smooth muscle. These drugs are to be used cautiously as they can precipitate arrhythmias (rhythm disturbances of heart) if taken in an over-dose in elderly patients with cardiac disease, hypertension, diabetes mellitus.

Cortico Steroids

a) Inhalational—budesonide, beclomethasone

b) Systemic—prednisolone, hydrocostisone

These drugs are potent anti-inflammatory drugs. They prevent release of phospholipids present in cell membranes. These phospholipids are converted (step by step) to prostoglandins and leukotriens which mediate inflammation. Corticosteroids also inhibit the release of various chemicals and factors which increase capillary permeability, contract smooth muscles and vasodilate. These corticosteroids also decrease mucosal oedema, bronchial hyperactivity and hypersecretion of mucus. Corticosteroids bring about both (1) symptomatic relief and (2) modify the disease. Oral therapy of corticosteroids is given for acute exacerbation of bronchial asthma.

Adverse Effects : Mouth and throat infections caused by *Candida albicans.*

Xanthine Derivatives

The drugs include aminophylline, theophylline, choline, theophillinate, etophylline. They inhibit a particular enzyme which by complex mechanisms brings about bronchodilatation. These drugs are used in bronchial and nocturnal asthma.

Mast Cell Stabilisation

The drugs include sodium oromoglycate ketotifen. These drugs exert their action by *'mast cell stabilisation'* and are considered important for prophylaxis (prevention) of asthma. Certain doctors do not agree with this view.

> Inhalers and spacers and nebulising solutions have all created revolution in the long-term management and treatment of asthma.

Drug Treatment of Asthma

Five or six years ago, managing one's asthma meant scrambling for a puff of bronchodilator as breathing suddenly became as arduous as sucking peanut butter through a straw. But lately, doctors have been abandoning this 'treat as needed' approach in favour of a preventive one, and while today's preventive treatment still targets the symptoms of asthma (inflammation and construction of the bronchial tubes) scientists are in hot pursuit of drugs that target the causes; the hyper-reactivity of those airways. Until the new drugs arrive, however, doctors should educate patients on how best to cope with existing therapies.

The first step in preventing attacks is to eliminate 'asthma triggers'. As discussed, skin tests can tell what triggers inflammation and bronchial constriction in a patient.

The next step is to determine how severe the disease is. Someone who experiences no symptoms other than tightness in the chest after, say, sprinting for the school bus, is a mild case and can usually get away with just a puff of a Bronchodilator before exercise. But an asthmatic who regularly wheezes needs a vertibale toolbox of drugs and devices starting with the inhaler.

Inhalers hold a cartridge that, when pressed, release a mist of medication. Another gadget is a 'peak flow meter' that measures the rate at which the lungs expel air into a tube. This is useful in calculating the amount of drug to be taken daily. It is a small tube-like apparatus that the patient blows through the tube, and it measures the force of his blow. That figure reveals how open the airways are and thus whether the patient needs a dose of medicine and, if so, which one and how much of it. Depending on the severity of the disease an asthmatic might use the monitor up to three times a day. In the more hightech models now available abroad a memory chip records the readings, and every month the patient downloads the numbers into a doctor's computer via a phone jack by monitoring the data. Physicians can the fine tune the treatment.

Drugs prescribed these days include Controllers and Relievers.

Relievers such as the inhalant, Albuterol, sold as ventolin and proventil, relax smooth muscles in the airways within seconds. They are, however, emergency measures.

Controllers include anti-inflammatories such as corticosteroids marketed as Vaneeril, Azmacort, and Flovent. Inhaled corticosteroids reduce inflammation in several ways including by interference with lung cells' secretion of Cytokines. These substances inflame the airways causing swelling and hence troubled breathing. Another anti-inflammatory Cromolyn Sodium (marketed as Intal) is less effective than steroids but is often prescribed for children because it is so safe. The other class of controllers is Bronchodilators like Salmeterol and Theophylline. They relax the lungs and keep the airways open.

Peak Flow Meter

Pollution, changes in lifestyle and various other factors are cited as the reasons for increase in the incidence of asthma. A peak flow meter monitors a patient's asthma the way a blood pressure cuff monitors the blood pressure. Peak flow is the measurement of how effectively the air moves out of one's lungs. Measuring peak flow helps determine any narrowing in one's airways before he has an actual attack. This allows him to take his medicine before a serious attack actually develops. It also helps in the adjustment of daily medication for asthma. So a peak flow meter can be an important part of our asthma management plan. Other benefits of peak flow monitoring include the following:

1) Helps him decide whether his condition is serious enough to seek emergency treatment.
2) Allows him to detect early stages of airway obstruction to start immediate treatment.
3) Gives one an accurate picture of the variations in his condition over a 24-hour period.
4) This permits his doctor to prescribe treatment when he needs it the most.
5) Helps him differentiate between airway obstruction and other causes of breathlessness like hyperventilation.
6) Allows him to ascertain specific allergens, irritants, or workplace exposures that may cause the symptoms to develop.
7) It can also act as an effective detector to monitor whether his asthma symptoms have stabilised, improved or deteriorated.

Peak flow meter needs care and cleaning. Dirt collected in the meter may make one's flow measurements inaccurate. If one has a cold or other respiratory infection, germs or mucus can also get collected in the meter.

Proper cleaning with a mild detergent in hot water will keep one's peak flow meter working accurately and may keep one using it healthier. Peak flow meters are available from Rs. 500/- onwards.

Imagine struggling to fill your lungs with air but not being able to get a deep breath. To some people, it sounds like a bad dream. For millions of others who have asthma, it is a common reality. For them, the 'medicinal inhalers' are literal lifesavers that restore breathing in 5-10 minutes by keeping airways open or opening blocked passages.

Asthma medications are grouped into categories : (1) anti-inflammatories which *reduce the risk of attack* and have to be taken regularly and (2) bronchodilators which stop or *control an attack* in progress. Inhalers are an excellent way to deliver both types of medication. They work quickly and have few side effects. However, *over use* of bronchodilators may make some people's asthma worse.

A patient taking inhaled steroids should use a spacer and clean it after every use. After using the inhaler, particularly one containing Corticosteroids, he must brush his teeth or rinse his mouth and spit out the water to prevent overgrowth of yeast.

Rotahalers

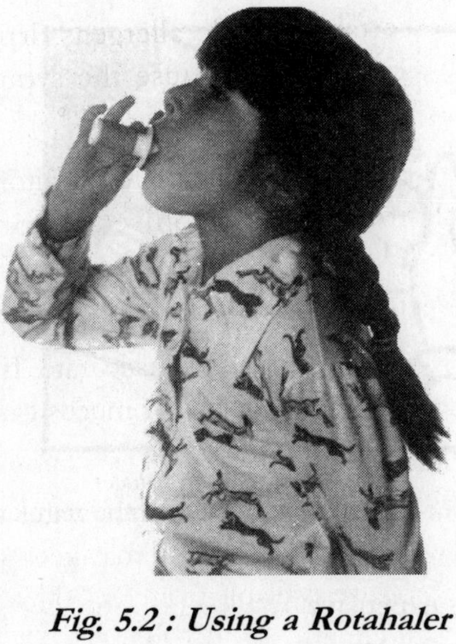

Fig. 5.2 : Using a Rotahaler

They are also available for use by asthmatics. Rotacaps of Asthalin, Beclate, Aerocort, Seroibid are all available which can be used in Rotahalers.

Spacer is a device to be used with metered dose inhalers. It helps solve the coordination problems and also enhances the deposition of the drug in lungs. It also reduces the oropharyngeal deposition and thus decreases the side effects.

How to use the Inhaler

1) Shake the inhaler vigorously.
2) Tilt your head back and breathe out.
3) Hold the inhaler either in the mouth or one inch from the mouth.
4) Activate the spray and inhale deeply and slowly.
5) Hold the breath for 10 seconds.
6) Wait for a minute.
7) Repeat all the above steps for subsequent puffs.

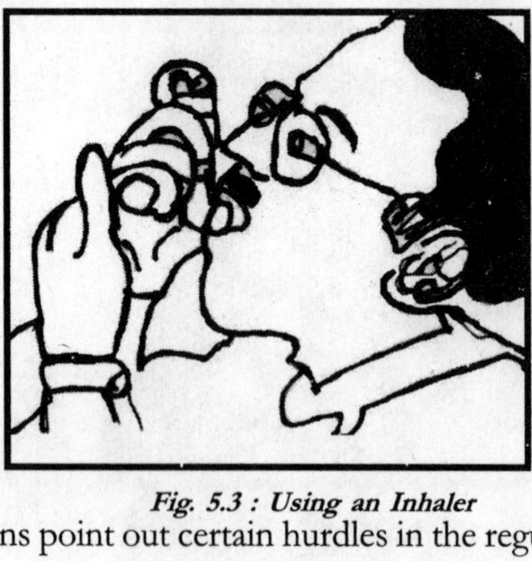

Fig. 5.3 : Using an Inhaler

Physicians point out certain hurdles in the regular use of steroid inhalers :

1) These are expensive.
2) There tends to be poor patient compliance.
3) Inhalers work very slowly, taking 10 days for any improvement to show.

4) It may appear to patients used to getting instant relief with sympathomimetic inhalers that these inhalers are not effective.

A Weekly Self Assessment Chart can be maintained by asthmatic patients. They can evaluate the symptoms (like coughs, wheeze and breathlessness) and also make a note of tablets/ injections they take, of the bronchodilator, steroids, theophyllines and antibiotic capsules per week. They can see how their symptoms are and how much they have to get medicated. If their symptoms are less, they take only few tablets and avoided steroids, injections, etc., that means they are improving. On the other hand, if their symptoms are on the increase, they are getting medicated with more and more injections and steroids as they are doing badly. This kind of self assessment aids in 'prognosis' by the patient himself.

A 'new controller' acts before a patient senses that an asthma attack is imminent. Leukotriene pathway inhibitors block the action of molecules that cause inflammation and constriction of the airways. Accolate and Syflo, approved in the USA in 1996, are the first offerings in this new category. Both are taken orally.

The majority of adult cases of asthma do not respond to anti-histamine drugs. In fact, in some cases, the symptoms tend to get aggravated with anti-histamines. But these drugs do provide relief to the children with allergic cough.

Given a choice asthmatics would just as soon decline the honour of having a newly fascinating disease, but the mysterious rise in the number of asthmatics may have a silver lining. It has set off a race to bring new asthma treatments to market. The biotech firm Genentech is testing a molecule that blocks the action of immunoglobulin E (IgE), an antibody produced in response to asthma triggers. As any sufferer knows IgE may be trying valiantly to fight off these invaders, but the collateral damage is huge. IgE binds to mast cells in the lungs and causes them to burst releasing histamine and other inflammatory molecules. Genentechs IgE inactivator is probably only a few steps away from market.

Fast acting relievers are being improved too. The leading one, Albuterol, is a mix of two mirror image molecules. The good twin opens up breathing passages. The evil twin can make kids hyper or nervous or cause irregular heart beat or insomnia. One way to avoid the effects of bad twin is to use a 'spacer' device in the inhaler to send the medicine to the back of the throat and lungs, keeping it away from the tongue where it can be swallowed and enter the bloodstream. One drug firm has another idea. It is trying to chemically separate out the bad twin leaving the molecule that dilates the airways. The drug will be out in the market soon or it is already out in the market; the rapid progress in medical pharmacology can achieve anything with lightning speed. This could be one of it.

Asthma Management Kits

In order to manage the asthma, pharmaceutical companies bring out many asthma management kits. These are useful both for the doctors and patients.

The kit includes :

1) Peak Flow Meter

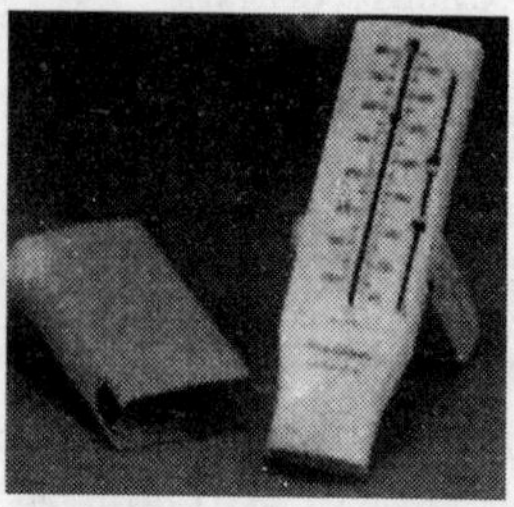

These are available as slimine, light-weight design meters with the unique thee zone-integrated asthma management system to get the precise and accurate peak flow expiratory rate (PEFR).

2) Drug Delivery System for Use with Metered Dose Inhalers.

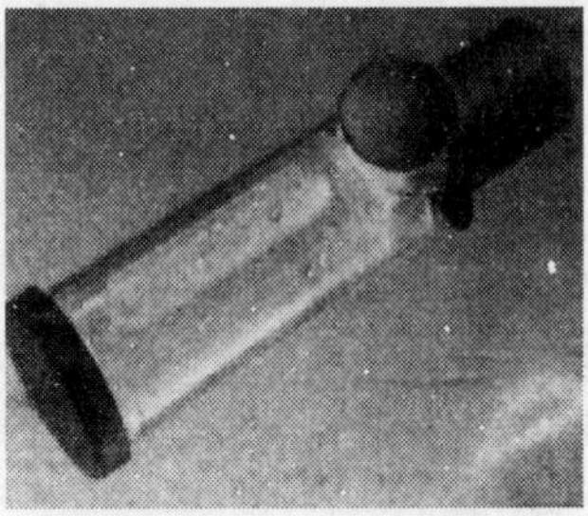

They are available in improved and easier-to-use design. The drug delivery system is a blend of spacer and metered dose inhaler with a special advanced feature of 'Aerosolisation'.

3) Inspiratory Muscle Trainers

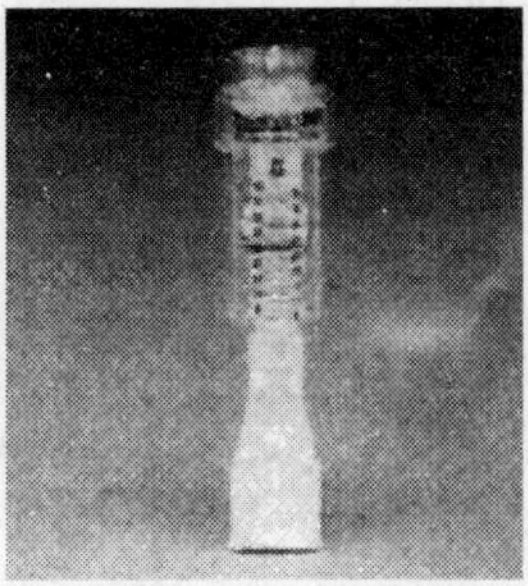

Certain models of these ensure constant inspiratory pressure load. The inspiratory lung muscle trainer is an exercise instrument for the lungs and is independent of the air flow and breathing rate.

These asthma management kits promise to improve the quality of life in the patient's suffering from asthma. With rapid progress happening in the field of asthma research, management, treatment, more and more sophisticated asthma management kits are likely to hit the market soon for the benefit of both the patients and the doctors who have to take care of their patients.

Today's asthma therapies are more effective than the increasing number of asthma cases suggests. The drugs, devices, precautions all work, but many patients, or in the case of children, their parents do not! With such patients in mind, researchers in the USA have created a molecule that strikes the very core of asthma. The exaggerated reactivity makes an asthmatic's airways inflamed and constricted in response to triggers that do not bother a non-asthmatic's lungs at all. This Antisense molecule deactivates the gene that produces the protein responsible for the hyper-reactivity.

Before discussing hyposensitisation two things are to be discussed very briefly :

1) Safety of Steroids

Short-term use of corlicosteroids has proved very helpful to those asthma patients who do not do well with bronchodilators. Time and dosage for which these steroids are given are within safe limits and have no serious side effects.

2) Status Asthmatics

Continuous and severe attack of asthma for more than 24 hours is called Status Asthmatics. This is an emergency condition. IV fluids, oxygen, corticosteroids, adrenaline and aminophylline all form an important part of treatment in this condition.

We will now discuss the hyposensitisation technique or immunotherapy. Once the diagnosis of extrinsic (allergic/atopic) asthma is made and the allergen involved is identified, two steps are to be followed immediately by the patient :

1) Avoid the thing the patient is allergic to.

2) If the allergen is a pollen, mould or dust present in the air and cannot be avoided the patient must be made resistant to the allergens.

Making the patient resistant to an allergen or allergens is done by a process called hyposensitisation or immunotherapy. The patient is injected with gradually increasing dose and concentrations of the extracts of the substances to which he is sensitive.

We have already discussed in detail how the extracts are made (refer skin tests). These extracts are given as injections to the patients. The three methods of hyposensitisation are:

1) *Pre-seasonal :* This is started three to four months prior to the onset of the season in which the patient gets the symptoms. Optimum dose is reached via injections before the offending season begins. Pre-seasonal injections are to be terminated at the onset of the season if the patient shows improvement or treatment can continue during the season (seasonally). During the season, the dose is reduced (because patient is inhaling allergen from air also and we cannot add to it by our treatment). Usually 15-20 injections constitute 1 pre-seasonal dose.

2) *Co-seasonal :* Injections are give to patients who present themselves during the pollen season.

3) *Perennial :* This consists of continuing the hyposensitisation even after the aggravating season. Injections are given throughout the year at intervals and spaced in evenly increasing periods.

Regarding schedules of injections, dilutions, etc., first very dilute extracts are given and later concentration is increased. The dose is also increased gradually. Some patients, as a result of the injection, complain of aggravation of their symptoms for a day or so. If aggravation of symptoms is unbearable, the dose is reduced. Most doctors believe that perennial therapy gives the maximum relief among the three methods of hyposensitisation.

The results of hyposensitisation as perceived by different doctors is different. Some doctors have claimed complete cure with hyposensitisation and others have claimed very poor results with it. There is no set standard for this method. The quality of extracts also varies from one place to another, dosage schedule also varies from one place to another. Accurate statistics on its efficacy is hence not available. The mechanism of hyposensitisation was once considered as blocking of antibodies against extracts to which the patient is allergic but this theory has failed as improvement in symptoms and blocking antibodies levels do not go hand in hand. 'Antigen Injection Mixtures' are prepared according to the allergy skin of the individual and is *special* for each patient. Injections are given in the upper arm, under the skin. The doctor decides the dose, concentration, etc. Injections are to be given regularly. The patient is carefully monitored. This is quite beneficial. Some local reaction like redness can occur but it is negligeble.

Hyposensitisation charts are maintained for each patient. It has the following columns:

Hyposensitisation Chart

Name of the patient .... Date ....

Date	*Dose and Concentration*	*Patient's Condition*	*Drugs taken*

Both the doctor and the patient involved in hyposensitisation should follow the schedule and record the data in the chart. Injection of antigen mixture should always be checked for dose, concentration and for quality. Contamination is to be strictly avoided. If the patient develops any local reaction, he can go ahead with the technique, but general reactions are to be taken as danger signals. It should be prevented at any cost and if it develops, he must be treated with adrenaline, antihistamines, oxygen, etc., as an emergency condition.

Make Your Home Asthma-Proof

Researchers suspect that allergens must be avoided to prevent asthma. Minimising homegrown triggers will help control symptoms.

(a) *Get rid of pets* : That includes cats, dogs, rabbits, guinea pigs. Animal dander is one of the top triggers. Getting rid of pet is non-negotiable. Let the critters be kept outside at least or in non-carpeted areas of the house such as kitchen.

(b) *Attack the dustmites :* It is not dust itself that causes the trouble but these microscopic pests. Carpets, bedding, upholstery and stuffed animals are their breeding grounds. Try hardwood floors and chairs. Cover pillows and mattresses with plastic casing, wash lines in hot water.

(c) *Declare war on cockroaches :* The bodies of dead cockroaches decompose and roach proteins waft through the house. Exterminate first, then scrub surfaces to eliminate any remains.

(d) *Control indoor moulds :* A dehumidifier is a good start. Zap bathroom mildew and get rid of fabrics in damp basements.

Summary

1) Diagnosis is by history, signs, symptoms, skin and inhalation tests.
2) Once the diagnosis of asthma is established medical treatment begins.
   a) Drugs used are controllers, relievers.
   b) Relievers relax smooth muscles.
   c) Controllers have anti inflammatavies such as corticosteroids. Cromolyn Sodium is another inflammatory less effective than steroids.
   d) Antihistamines are useful only in allergic cough in children.

   e) Bronchodilators are another class of controllers that relax lungs and keep airway open.

   f) Inhalers, peak flow meters are excellent gadgets for drug delivery.

3) Hyposensitisation is increasing resistance to allergen. Its efficacy ranges from 'complete cure' to 'No use at all'.

6

ASTHMA : FACTS AND MYTHS

Fact Sheet for Asthmatics

1) Asthma has existed since early times because the very name of the disease comes from a Greek word that means 'Panting or gasping for breath'.

2) The incidence of asthma is higher in congested and crowded urban areas.

3) Male children are more prone to asthma than female children. However, the gap becomes negligible after the first 12 years. In adults, it is equal in both sexes.

4) Asthmatic attacks tend to come suddenly. The most severe attacks can be controlled temporarily. There are drugs that can effectively relieve an acute attack.

5) People of any age can have asthma but at least 50 per cent cases are between 20 and 40.

6) The factors that precipitate an attack of asthma are acute respiratory tract infection, exposure to one of the allergens, exertion, sudden change in temperature and emotional stress.

7) The most common symptoms of asthma are wheezing, a hard, dry cough, a sense of suffocation, inability to expel air easily from lungs.

8) In an acute asthmatic attack, hospitalisation is often necessary to prevent suffocation.

9) The most common time for an attack to occur is early morning hours or during the night.

10) Asthma like allergies is not contagious.

11) Asthma is almost never fatal unless left untreated.

12) Nervousness never causes asthma but there is a definite relationship between the two.

13) An asthmatic can lead the life like any other normal person by taking proper measures. He can prevent the occurrence of attacks.

14) Emotional factors are known to be quite an important factor affecting asthmatic patients. Asthma can lead to severe psychological disturbances in the family.

Allergy—Facts

There has been a steady increase in the number of persons affected by allergy and immunological disorders in India. Every year the survey shows that there has been an increase in the population affected by allergies. This can be attributed to environmental pollution, urbanisation and an increase in cheap, substandard cosmetic and food products in the consumer markets. Recent studies suggest allergies affect the brain and the nervous system leading to symptoms, like :

1) headaches
2) depression
3) nervousness
4) hyperactive states
5) convulsions
6) nocturnal eneurises (bed wetting)
7) disturbances of urinary bladder.

Asthma Facts

Medical researchers have observed that in some patients, breathlessness is primarily caused by heart disease. This condition also occurs due to mental fatigue and depression. *Cardiac Asthma* is a common feature in a case of hypertensive heart disease and coronary artery disease.

Cortisone and allied drugs have proved valuable in providing immediate relief to asthma patients and for short-term treatment. But their long-term use does have side effects.

Hysterical Asthma—Some patients, particularly young girls, complain of 'Asthma like' symptoms. However, there are no signs of wheeze or breathlessness. All they have is what is called *Sighing Respiration.*

Myths about Asthma

Myth 1 : Children outgrow their asthma.

Parents tend to believe that with growth and maturity the problems of children get sorted out. Children with mild symptoms may in rare cases outgrow asthma. However, it is quite difficult to segregate such cases. The prevalence of asthma among children is higher than among adults. According to available data, nearly 10 per cent of the children below 12 years of age and 5 per cent of adults have this disease.

Myth 2 : Asthma can cause tuberculosis or lung cancer.

There is no medical evidence to support this common misconception. Perhaps, the intense discomfort experienced by asthmatic patients lead them to assume that something more disastrous is in store for them.

Myth 3 : Nasal allergy and asthma have little connection.

About 40 per cent of patients who have nasal allergy develop asthma. The lining of the nose continues into the bronchial tubes. Asthma in most cases is because of nasal allergy being passed into them. The same irritants that cause swelling and excessive secretion in the lining of the nose produce similar results in the lining of the bronchial tubes. The bronchial tube passages become narrower because of swelling of their linings, contraction of the muscle tissues in the bronchial walls, or from plugging with thick mucus. These cause difficulty in breathing and induce coughing attacks, the major symptoms of asthma.

Myth 4 : Taking vitamins can cure asthma.

What is required is not vitamins but well known drugs that can effectively relieve an asthamatic attack. Vitamins are largely prescribed for curing deficiencies, they cannot cure asthma. Perhaps, their value is more psychological.

Myth 5 : Change of climate cures asthma.

It does not. But it may be valuable if the allergic causes of asthma are not present in the new location. Patients who are helped by warm, dry, equitable climate are those whose disease is primarily due to chronic bronchial infection. But asthma in children is rarely helped by change of climate. Sometimes a child is relieved by an escape to a new environment. But it has been seen that the patient develops 'sensitivity' to the allergens in two to three years in his new environment.

Myth 6 : Emotional tension causes asthma.

Emotional tension alone is rarely the major cause of the patient's trouble. It may, however, aggravate the condition and make the patient more prone to asthma attacks. Asthma can produce a variety of abnormal changes and responses. Emotions such as anxiety, fear, anger and strong excitement can cause an allergic attack. But there will always be a physical basis for the allergy.

Myth 7 : Asthma is a precursor to heart problems.

Medical evidence does not support this widely propagated misconception. The difficulty in breathing leads to fears of heart attacks. The increased strain of the repeated attacks may have an adverse effect on the heart. This takes a long time, however, and is not a very common occurrence.

Summary

1) We have learnt interesting facts and figures about asthma.
2) We have discussed the myths about asthma.

7

ASTHMA, TONSILS AND ADENOIDS

Asthma among Children

The course and severity of asthma among children are difficult to predict. The majority of affected children have occasional attacks of slight to moderate severity, which is not very difficult to manage. A minority of them develop severe intractable asthma, usually perennial rather than seasonal. It is this that is traumatic as it can be incapacitating and adversely affects school attendance, day-to-day functioning and general child activity.

First Symptoms

Thirty per cent of patients are symptomatic in their first year of life. About 85 per cent of the asthmatic children have their first symptoms before four to five years age. Most affected children are likely to experience wheezing during the first year, especially where there is a family history of asthma and other allergic diseases. Such children could show signs of growth retardation.

Prognosis

This is generally encouraging for young asthmatic children. Ultimately remission depends partly upon growth in the cross-sectional diameter of the airway. About 50 per cent of all asthmatic children are virtually free of symptoms within 10-20 years, but recurrences are common in adulthood. In children, who have mild asthma with onset between two years and puberty, the remission rate is almost 50 per cent and only 5 percent develop severe disease. In contrast, children with chronic steroid dependent disease with frequent hospitalisation rarely improve and 95 per cent such cases become adult asthmatics. Quick and fast diagnosis and treatment are needed to control asthmatic attacks in children. Medical experts say that among factors that put the children in the high risk category are : underestimation of the severity of the illness by the family or physician leading to a delay in treatment, under-use of steroids and non-compliance of the prescribed treatment.

Experts classify asthmatic patients into three types—mild, moderate or severe, based on the history, physical examination, lab data and need for medication. Children with mild asthma have attacks of varying frequency, up to once each week. The attacks are not severe and the child responds to branchodilator treatment in one or two days. Generally, medication is not required between attacks when the child is essentially free of symptoms of airway obstruction. Children with mild asthma have good school attendance, exercise tolerance and are largely able to get uninterrupted sleep. Children with moderate asthma, however, show these same symptoms more frequently. They cough more often and have mild wheezing between more severe exacerbations. School attendance is irregular, exercise tolerance is less due to coughing and wheezing and sleep is disturbed. They need regular and continuous medical attention rather than intermittent bronchodilator therapy.

Severe Asthma

This needs to be recognised early. Such children have virtually daily wheezing and more frequent and more severe exacerbations. Recurrent hospitalisation is often necessary. They have poor school attendance, unsound sleep and poor exercise tolerance. Due to their chronic hyper-inflation, they develop chest deformities. Continuous and systemic medical treatment is required. During severe attacks, round-the-clock therapy is necessary to achieve adequate control of the illness.

Asthma in Older People

Asthma manifests itself differently in children, adults and elderly people. In children it is usually manifested as cough and wheeze; in adults as paroxysmal attacks of breathlessness; in older people, while paroxysmal attacks may continue, exertional dyspnoea (breathlessness on exertion) also set in due to the complications of chronic bronchitis and emphysema. While adult asthma patients feel normal in between the attacks, older patients continue getting breathlessness on exertion even while they do not have the asthma attack.

Those who first get asthma in their old age are far worse than those who have had the onset in their youth. Treatment of asthma in older patients needs much more attention and care. Male patients having enlarged prostrate gland face a particular difficulty. Administration of bronchodilators containing ephedrine may lead to hesitancy in passing urine or lead to the retention of urine.

Corticosteroids can lead to osteoporosis and fracture of fragile bones. The incidence of tuberculosis is also appreciable in those who take corticosteroids. Adrenaline given during status asthmaticus endangers the heart and blood vessels of those who have hypertensive heart disease.

Enlarged Adenoids and Tonsils in Asthma

Tonsils and adenoids are lymphoid tissues present in the neck. They defend the body against germs or other dangerous substances that try to enter our body through the mouth or nose. They produce antibodies which circulate in the body and fight the intruders which have entered the body by passing the tonsils. Tonsils enlarge unduly in some children in the process of protecting the body from germs. Whether the enlarged tonsil is to be removed is a big controversial question. There are three views regarding whether the tonsils have to be removed or not in a child with allergic manifestations such as cough and wheeze.

1) Tonsils act initially as the site and subsequently as a source of infection in the body. So its *removal is favourable* in the course of asthma and also prevents its occurrence in a susceptible individual.

2) Tonsils prevent the spread of infection from the nose and throat to the lungs and bronchi. Therefore, their removal will make a mild asthmatic attack into a severe one or might even cause an asthmatic attack in a susceptible individual. Thus, *removal is harmful.*

3) Absence or presence of tonsils has no effect on the allergic status of an individual. The removal of tonsils or retaining them can neither cause an attack nor can prevent an attack. It has a *neutral approach.*

Location of the Tonsils and Adenoids

Allergic children are more susceptible to infections of the chest and throat. If evidence of infection in the throat exists and if the infection localised in the tonsils appear again and again, the tonsils need to be removed, but with the understanding that it has no effect on asthma which the child is suffering from. Tonsillectomy does not do anything to the 'Allergic Entity' in children causing asthma. In some cases benefits of tonsillectomy was found greater in the first post-operative year than in the second.

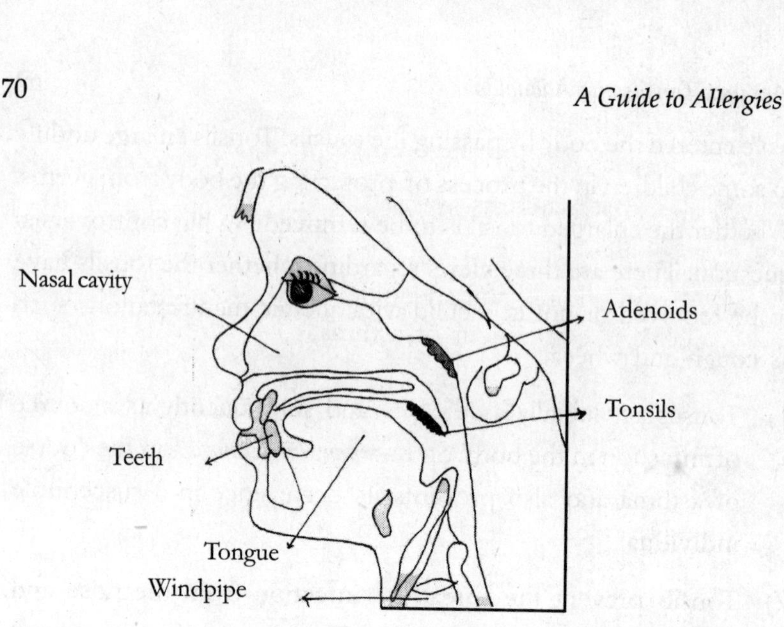

Fig. 7.1 : Location of the Tonsils in the Body

Improvement in symptoms must have increased (and not decreased) if tonsillectomy had anything to do with asthma. Tonsillectomy indications are the same for both asthmatic and non-asthmatic children. The indications are (1) chronic infections of tonsils and adenoids (2) marked enlargement of tonsils and adenoids causing interference in breathing and swallowing and (3) recurrent ear infections.

The discussion above holds good for adenoids and adenoidectomy also which need not be discussed separately. Thus, an asthmatic child with enlarged tonsils has to be evaluated for allergy like any other asthmatic child, and the allergy has to be treated. Removal of tonsils has nothing to do with allergy.

Summary

1) Pediatric asthma has got certain special features.

2) Classification of asthma into mild, moderate, severe type is done on the basis of history, physical examination, lab

test findings and the need for medication.

3) Asthma manifests as Exertional dysphora in geriatric age group.

4) Tonsillectomy and adenoidectomy have no effect on the allergic component of asthma.

8

LIFESTYLE CHANGES IN ASTHMA

Non-drug treatment (NDT) is neither new nor revolutionary, but a number of case studies have shown that NDT has resulted in patients reporting an improved quality of life and more self-confidence. This is not to say that medication can be avoided totally. But NDT perhaps offers a more holistic approach to managing asthma. The hitch is that NDT requires hard work on the part of both the patient and the physician. One of the main benefits of NDT is that there is a marked drop in the consumption of drugs, and a reduced need for steroids and antibiotics which is both medically and psychologically beneficial to the patient in the long run. The main pillars of NDT are (1) knowledge of disease (2) allergy control (3) diet (4) changes in daily routine (5) exercise and (6) management of psychological factors.

1. Knowledge of Disease

Throughout the world people are suffering asthmatic reactions to a range of allergens that once caused little trouble. Though scientists are learning more about asthma, its increasing incidence is still a mystery. In the course of a few decades what was once an obscure allergic syndrome has emerged as one of the most vexing health problems. The number of asthma sufferers has jumped by over 60 per cent since the early 1980's and the death toll is also increasing.

The patient should have thorough knowledge of the disease. The dynamics of asthma are no mystery. The trouble starts when the immune system becomes sensitised to some allergens. Whenever the irritant enters the body the immune system's beta cells (lymphocytes) produce a lot of anti-body molecules IgE. There attach to antigen, then from a complex, trigger most calls to produce histamine etc. which bring about inflammation and the cascade of events continue bringing an attack. This concept must be clearly explained to the patient.

Anything can act as an irritant. Toddlers who live with smokers are three times more likely to wheeze as kids in smoke free homes. Dustmites that thrive on carpet, bedding leave behind a highly allergenic protein. All these points must be understood by the patient. Asthma is not usually a problem in pre-industrial societies regardless of the national surroundings. But when development sets in, asthma quickly follows.

In an 1991 study of children in Zimbabwe it was found that only one in 1,000 of those living in rural villages suffered from obstructed airways but asthma plagued one in 17 of those in the prosperous section of capital, Harare. Researchers have documented the same pattern among the urban population in countries like Kenya, South Africa, Papua New Guinea, New Zealand and Australia. Even within the Western counties increasing urbanisation sees people more and more vulnerable to this condition.

The points mentioned above gives the patient an insight as to what he is suffering from, its magnitude, proportions and prevalence. The patient must understand the nature of the disease, allergic factors causing it, allergens, their role, how to avoid them, about signs/symptoms, medications, i.e., he must have an 'A to Z' knowledge of the diseases.

2. Allergy Control

A lot of discussion has been done regarding this aspect in previous chapters. Once the cause in found out and the effect in linked to the cause the main line of treatment will be to avoid the cause. We have discussed the ways to avoid various allergens, how to substitute them with something harmless or to develop resistance to it by hyposensitisation.

3. Diet

Recommended are green, leafy vegetables like spinach and fenugreek leaves (methi), fruits like papaya, chikoos, apples and mangoes, salads like beetroot and carrot, since these coloured fruits and vegetables contain a chemical called flavonoids that is anti-allergic in nature. Such a diet also takes care of constipation which is a minor trigger factor of asthma attacks. Equally beneficial is drinking a glass of hot water in the morning because it helps in loosening and drainage of the sputum. It is also advisable to drink plenty of water during the day and eat something frequently rather than have two or three heavy meals. It is a also not advisable for asthmatics to sleep after heavy meals. The dietary dont's for asthma patient include deep fried foods like somosa and puri, and sour foods like curds, tamaind, lassi, shrikand, etc. Also care should be taken to avoid bananas, raw onions, citrus fruits like mosambi, orange, lemon and grapes, cold foods like ice cream, kulfi. Cold drink should also be avoided.

On the whole the diet of an asthmatic should be light, nutritious, and well balanced. Most of the patients of asthma dont feel comfortable with lady'sfingers among vegetables and black gram (urad dal) among lentils. These can be avoided. Spices must also be avoided. Asthma patients should take more of vegetables, soups, fruits, all to be taken in moderation. Children need more carbohydrates and more proteins. They must avoid pickles, chuttnies, etc. Old people with asthma, especially those taking corticosteroids, may have osteoporosis. They need more of calcium, protein, vitamin, minerals, etc. Milk, soyabeans can be given in optimum quantities. If the elderly is a non-vegetarian he can take chicken soup, meat, egg, fish provided he is not allergic to any of them. Intake of fat should be limited. Multivitamin tablets with mineral should be added to the daily diet. Smoking and drinking are to be avoided by all asthmatics, irrespective of age and sex.

Basic Diet Rule for Asthmatics

'No' for
- Fried fatty foods
- Smoking/drinking
- Overloading stomach at nigh

'Yes' for
- Simple nutritious food
- light dinners
- Plenty of water during attacks

4. Changes in Daily Routine

Daily routine changes have to be made in an asthmatic patient. These include:

i) *Regular Routine*

Regularity must be followed in diet, work, etc. This reduces symptoms in an asthmatic. Any irregularity in this diet, work, sleeping and working hours affect them badly. Regularity in daily routine is very essential for an asthma patient. He must go to bed and get up in the morning at regular times. He can go for a walk in the morning or do some physical workout at home. He should take a simple diet at regular hours.

ii) *Avoidance of Smoking*

An asthma patient should not smoke at all. Smoke and Smoky particles are irritants to the respiratory tract and produce both bronchospasm and respiratory infection.

iii) *Avoidance of Hard Drinks*

Drinking causes irregularities in diet or overeating. This may predispose to an attack of asthma, hence drinking in best avoided.

iv) *Cleanliness*

Keeping the bedroom clean is very important for an asthmatic. He must avoid cluttering his bedroom with a lot of things. No rugs or carpet, the furniture should be simple and the room must be cleaned daily. The bedroom should also be protected from extraneous disturbing sounds.

(v) *Avoidance of Air Pollution*

Air pollution has to be avoided as far as possible. Outings and picnics in places like gardens/ countryside are best avoided as they may precipitate symptoms in him. The residence and place of profession must be chosen avoiding all the allergy- triggering factors.

(vi) *Diet Regimen*

The patient should use his discretion and regulate his food habits according to his symptoms. After all, the life of an asthmatic patient in not a life in an 'army camp'. He can also indulge a little bit in his food habit when it is a symptom-free season.

(vii) *Medication*

Proper intake of medicines and tablets should be practised. He should consult a doctor if there is any doubt. If he has no doubt he can follow the drug regime carefully by himself.

Sports and Asthmatics

Most asthmatics can safely swim (lots of warm, moist air to breathe). Even gymnastics are usually all right (lots of stops and starts). Track and basketball are riskier. Soccer is fine for kids whose symptoms are controlled by a puff of ventolin before kickoff. For more severe cases, playing full back or as a goalie is safer than a forward.

> **Asthma**
>
> 'It can be Beaten.'
>
> The three golden rules are:
>
> 1) know the warning signs.
>
> 2) always keep medication handy.
>
> 3) make your home allergy free.

An exercise prescription for asthmatics is:

Work out to Reduce Risks.

Asthma we all know in characterised by narrowing of air passages within the bronchial tubes and lungs and this causes wheezing and chest tightness. It has the potential to lead to shortness of breath and respiratory failure. Young children suffer the most from asthma in units with rampant air pollution. The condition can also be progressive and serious for adults. As per the latest research asthma has been linked to allergies, immune disorders and a new generation of drugs which work to dilate passage ways without increasing the heart rate. Exercise is very important in asthmatics. Many famous athletes have asthma but have learned to train and perform well under pressure. Often they start out by producing relaxation techniques concentrating on practising inhalation and exhalation in a calm manner. They also learn pursed lip breathing which provides a subtle back pressure on the airways with the result of keeping the alveoli of bronchiol tube callapsing. The best type of exercise for asthma sufferers is aerobics. It helps to open the lungs, slightly increase lung volume, increase the capacity of the muscles to extract oxygen from the circulating blood and improve the body's ability to rid itself of toxic waste such as co_2 and lactic acid. The types of aerobic exercise can be everything from walking, slow jogging, swimming (but not in cold weather) and games such as cricket. In fact any intermittent aerobic activity that includes start and stop motion is ideal since the likelihood of inducing an asthma attack is reduced. Interspersing frequent brief rest periods with jogging, walking or rowing can be beneficial. People with asthma who are inhalers on bronchodilators should take two puffs before beginning exercise. This form of pre-medicating can reduce the sensitivity in the airways since exercise itself can sometimes create an allergic response within some individuals. Exercise is good medicine. A daily dose of it is the perfect percription whether for chronic medical condition or to enhance the general state of realth.

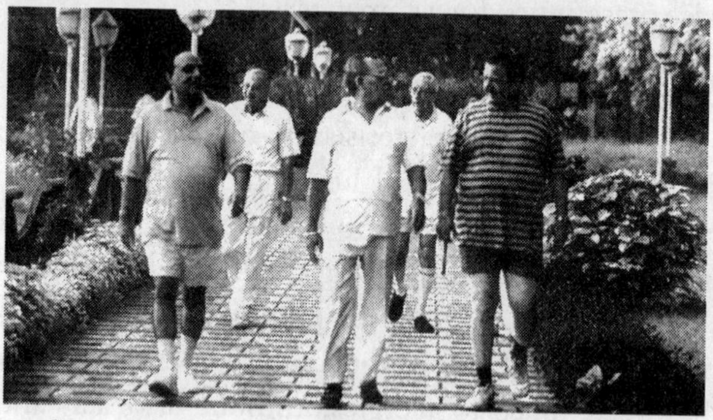

Not only regularity in physical activity but also regularity in mentioned activity is also important for an asthmatic. He must avoid tension and accumulating too much of work and decision making. He must also stop worrying over unwanted issues. Too much of mental tension can cause an attack of asthma.

5. Exercises for Asthma Patients

There are two types of exercises that are helpful for an asthma patient: breathing exercises to improve the condition of the lungs and exercises for general fitness. Breathing exercises include air pillow blowing and balloon blowing for about 10 minutes or bubbling into a bowl of water with a straw for five minutes or even playing a musical instrument like a flute or a mouth organ to improve lung power. Regular exercises facilitate drainage of infected sputum.

In normal breathing it is the diaphragm that does the greatest amount of work. When one inhales the diaphragm moves downward and when one exhales the diaphragm moves upward, squeezing the air out of the lungs.

The asthma patient over a period of time develops an unnatural habit of breathing during an attack. The tendency for him is to breathe mostly and quickly from the upper part of the chest rather than the whole chest. This makes the chest muscle work hard, particularly so as they are working against constricted airways.

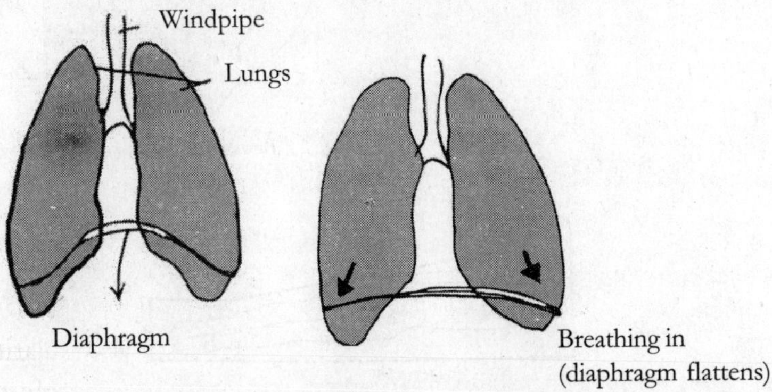

Fig. 8.1 : How the Diaphragm Works

Breathing exercises aim at:

i) Relaxing the overworked chest muscles.

ii) Increasing the use of diaphragm and of the abdominal muscle rather than the chest muscles.

In order to achieve the proper working of the diaphragm and lower chest the asthma patient has to concentrate on breathing out rather than breathing in. Breathing out has to be a slow process and not a hasty one as it may lead to wheezing and discomfort if done in a hurry. He must concentrate all his attention on pushing out his abdomen. This automatically leads to lower chest breathing.

The patient must try to empty his chest and raise the diaphragm by voluntary contraction of abdomen and lower chest

↓

This well reverse the procedure which exists during an asthmatic attack.

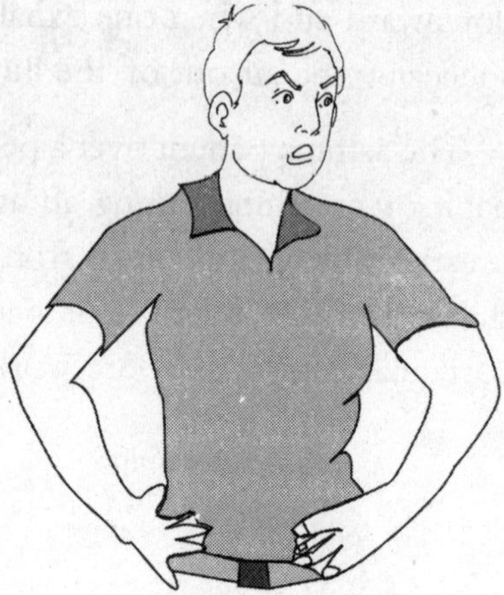

Fig. 8.2 : Breathing Exercises help in Asthma

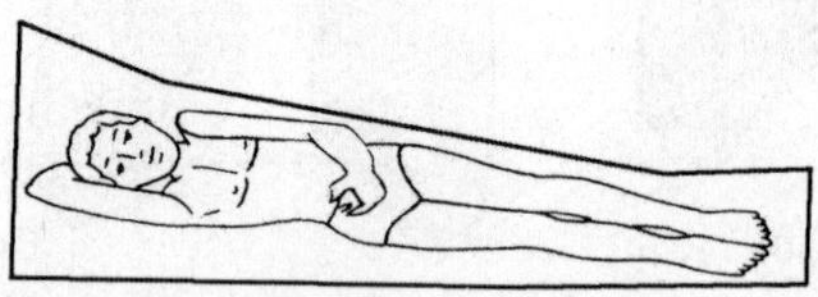

Fig. 8.3 : Comfortable Lying Position during an Asthma Attack

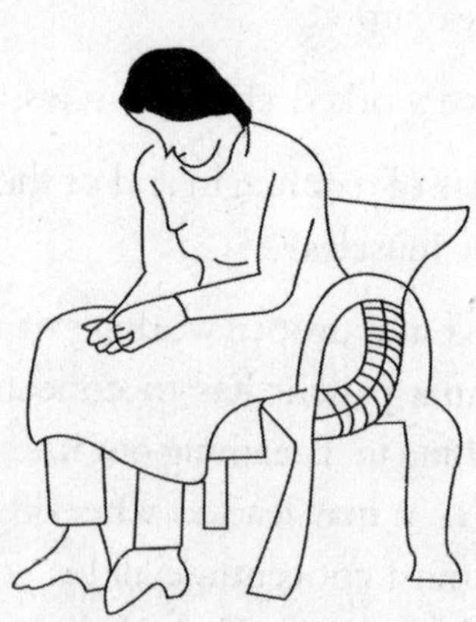

Fig. 8.4 : Comfortable Sitting Position during an Asthma Attack

Relaxation of the chest muscles: Relaxation of the body and the chest muscle from the first stage of this re-training programme can be achieved by different positions and exercises. One of them is explained below.

Sit with legs stretched and feet apart, arms hanging relaxedly on the sides. Breathe out slowly and drop the head until it reaches between the knees. Raise the body gradually until the lower part of the back is straight first, followed by the middle point of the back, upper part of the back, head. Keep breathing in until the starting position is reached. This exercise has to be done very slowly. This is called forward bending exercises. It can also be done in the standing position.

An important position particularly useful in an attack of asthma is to sit and lean forward with the head and arms resting on the pillows on a table. This "comfortable lying position" during an asthma attack its shown in figure 8.3.

'Forward Tilting of the trunk' is the key to all positions and exercises. Once the relaxation position is reached the patient's sequence of thoughts should be relaxation of hands, neck, chest and the maintenance of these while breathing rhythmically with his lower ribs.

Diaphragm and abdomina muscles exercises: These are different exercises and positions. If this is combined which the relaxed position already explained it can be very useful. Toe touching exercise, sit ups are all for using the diaphragm and abdominal muscles. The following diagrams below show how they are done. But *breathing out during the exercise* and *breathing in at rest* are the most important aspects of these exercises. They have to be done 10 times for optimum results. The exercise has to be done very slowly. No sudden or jerky movements. The muscles should not be tired.

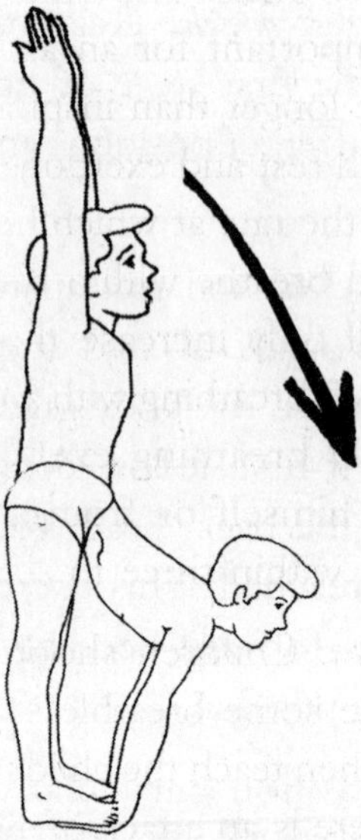

Fig. 8.5 : Toe Touching Exercise

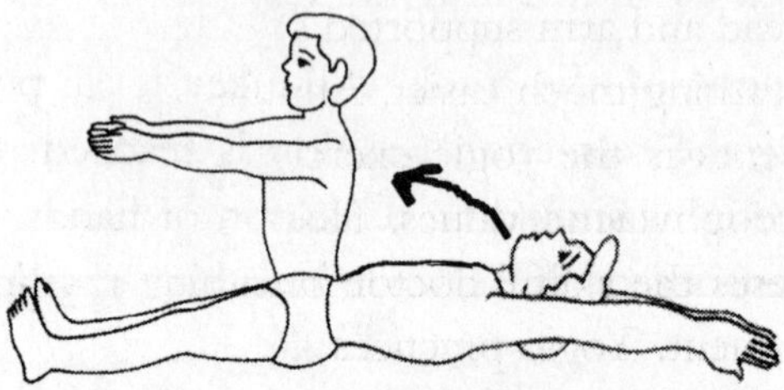

Fig. 8.6 : Sit-up Exercise

The exercises can all be repeated many times a day. A habit should be formed. When breathing in, the upper chest should be kept still so that breathing is performed by the diaphragm. When breathing out, the whole chest should relax. While doing the exercises the above points are to be followed. Breathing in is to be done through the nose and breathing out to be done through the mouth with a hissing sound.

Expiration-inspiration Ratio: The time taken for inspiration and expiration is very important for an asthmatic patient. Normally expiration should be longer than inspiration in the ratio of 3 : 2. This appears for both rest and exertion. The patient should try to fit in this rhythm to the rate at which he is breathing. When he is breathless, he should breathe within his wheeze. Any attempt to force expiration will only increase the wheeze and spasm. He should do gentle, quick breathing with a longer expiration reducing the speed. Gradually breathing exercises can be learnt by an asthmatic either by himself or from a physiotherapist. He can learn these exercises within three to six weeks.

Exercise for children: Children should be encouraged to play games. With exercise some breathlessness gets normal. Parents must first learn and then teach the child the techniques that should be adopted when there is an attack of breathlessness. A child can perform breathing exercises while lying down when there is breathlessness. Small children find it easy to sit on their heels and lean forward head and arm supported on a pillow. This makes the lower chest breathing much easier. Another form of exercise for asthmatic patients is the yogic exercises. Yogic practices have curative and prophylactic values. Health yoga pradipika states that in all diseases the skilful doctor must give scientific, medical and yogic treatment. Yogic practices are finding a lot of use in the treatment of asthma. The various techniques adopted are:

i) *Savasana* (corpse pose) which *prana dharana*

ii) *Makarasana* (crocodile pare)

Persons having a history of chronic colds and sinusitis are taught *neti kriya* (nose cleaning) with water and a rubber catheter. *Neti kriya* is done with salt water, milk and honey also. This procedure is said to develop resistance in the nasal mucous membrane to withstand variations in temperature and barometric pressure of the environment.

Neti kriya with milk is for developing resistance against proteins and with honey it is for developing resistance against pollens.

Persons having cough with expectoration are taught *Dhautis*.

This includes
- i) *Vara Dhauti* (cleaning with a cloth). This help to remove mucous secretions which are in excess in the stomach.
- ii) *Vaman danda* (cleaning with a stick).

For removal of sputum from the lungs *Kapalabhati kriya* (diaphragmatic breathing) in advocated.

Dhautis are very effective in the treatment of asthma. They are best suited in averting an attack of asthma. Yogic treatment reduces the quantity of drugs in persons suffering from chronic colds, sinusitis, bronchitis along with asthma. Though yogic procedures cannot bring about complete relief, they are important supportive treatment procedures that bring about improvement in symptoms.

Kapalabhati : The person sits in *Varjasana*. He must close the fingers of both the hands, keeping the thumb inside, and place them on his thighs, touching each other.

Inhalation and exhalation are performed with great vigour. Inhalation should be mild and slow, and long exhalation should be done quickly and forcibly by contracting the abdominal muscles with a backward push for as many as 60-80 times at a stretch.

There is *no retention* in this *Pranayama*.

It cleanses the respiratory system and nasal passages. Asthma is relieved. Carbon dioxide is eliminated and the heart functions better.

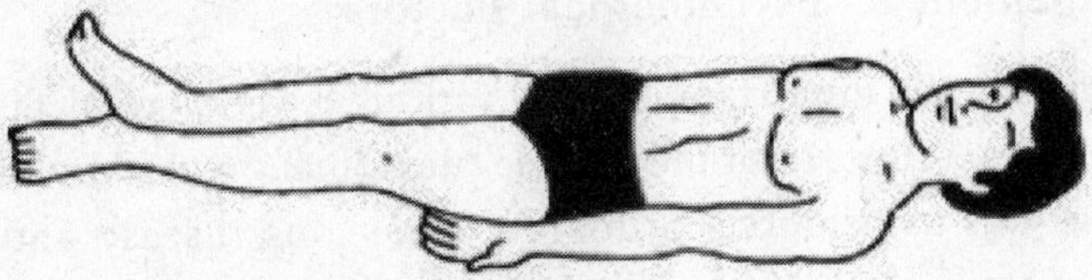

Fig. 8.7 : Savasana (Corpse pose)

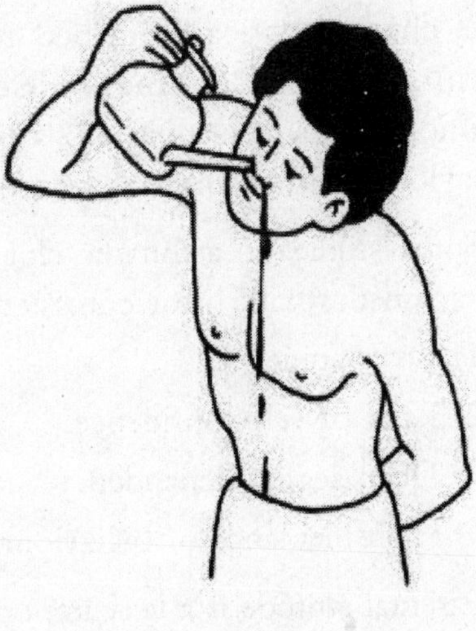

Fig. 8.8 : Jal Neti (Nose cleaning)

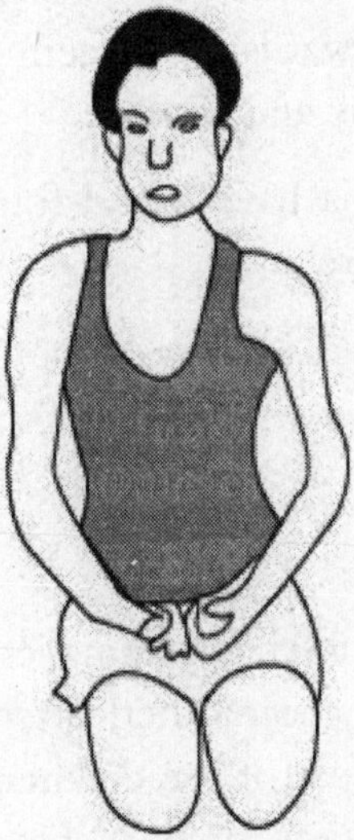

Fig. 8.9 : Kapalabhati

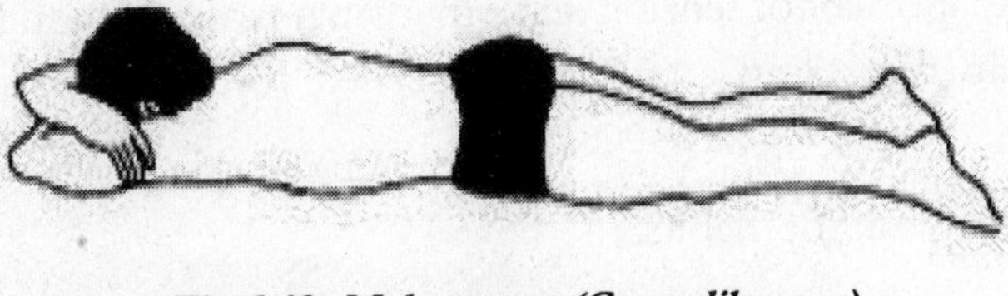

Fig. 8.10 : Makarasana (Crocodile pose)

Management of Psychological Factors

Asthma has an important link to various psychological factors. Once upon a time, until the allergic phenomenon was discovered asthma was considered primarily a nervous disease and was referred to as 'Asthma nervosa' in older textbooks of medicine.

In 1955, Dr. Bastiaans and Dr. Bren described many characteristics in the personality of the asthmatics. Out of the nine characteristics described three characteristic are often mentioned when asthma is discussed. They are (1) marked emotional hypersensitivity (2) a tendency towards domineering behaviour and (3) strong reactions of jealousy and rivalry.

Some studies in asthmatic children in India have found four characteristics with great consistency. They are :

1) Over-anxiety
2) Lack of self-confidence
3) Deep-seated dependency
4) High incidence of behaviour problems

Parental attitude is a very important factor in child asthmatics. Unsatisfactory parental attitude, especially of the mother, often causes or precipitates an attack of asthma. Most of the children who are asthmatic exhibit either fear and anxiety, or they show dependence or superego. Asthmatic attacks in children can get caused due to tension of examination. Fear of an asthma attack itself can trigger a attack. Tense patients must learn to relax. As far as management of tension and other such psychological factors which can trigger an attack is concerned four rules are to be followed:

1) Regular routine habits.
2) Morning walk/exercise; well balanced diet; regular hours of sleep and work.

3) Meditation, *Shavasana*, prayer or other relaxation techniques.

4) Avoiding excess work, tension and stress.

Accepting the situation is the most important rule for asthmatics. They need not fear their disease. Attacks can be prevented. Medical treatments are available for attacks if they happen. Once they practically approach their condition they will be tension-free and can then develop a relaxed mind.

Besides all this being part of support groups like the Asthma and Bronchitis Association of India and taking part in their various activities help greatly in cultivating a sense of belonging and self-confidence in patients.

Summary

1) NDT is Non-Drug Treatment.

2) The patient of asthma should take a simple, balanced and nutritious diet.

3) Breathing and yogic exercises are valuable supportive treatments.

4) A tension-free, relaxed mind helps in living with asthma.

5) Important lifestyle changes include:
   a) Regulation in day-to-day routine.
   b) Following the drug regime regularly.
   c) No smoking/alcohol.

6) *Acceptance* of the asthmatic condition is to live with it.

9

ALTERNATE SYSTEMS AND ASTHMA

Asthma — How Other Systems of Medicine View It

Before we discuss what the various alternate systems of medicine say about Asthma and how they approach it treatment wise, we will see in a *nutshell* what allopathy says about bronchial asthma.

Essence: Generalised airways obstruction which in the early stages at least is paroxysmal and reversible. Mucous membrane swelling, viscid mucus, and bronchial muscle contraction may cause obstruction.

History: Intermittent wheezing, dysphonia, cough. Precipitating causes can be anxiety, infections, exercise, allergen. A history of the patient may also reveal other allergic diseases (eczema) and asthma.

An examination of the patient reveals the following findings:

1) Audible wheeze on expiration;
2) Severe asthma is indicated by use of accessory muscles of respiration;
3) Difficulty in talking;
4) Tachycardia (high heart rate) or Bradycardia (low heart-rate)—this is worse;
5) Reduced breath sounds and cyanosis (bluish hue of skin); and

6) Pulsus Paradoxus (exaggerated decrease in systolic BP with inspiration; normal decrease is <10 mm of Hg).

Investigations to be done on an asthma patient depends on the severity :

1) Peak flow serial measurements (e.g., at home).
2) Chest x-ray (reveals pneumotherax (air in thorax- aspergillosis).
3) Complete blood count and sputum cytology reveal eosinophilia (i.e., raised eosonophil count) if any.
4) Prick tests (reveal allergens).
5) Measuring lung volumes indicate degree of obstruction.

Differential Diagnosis : Pulmonary oedema (cardiac asthma), chronic bronchitis (cough is present, obstruction is irreversible) and pneumothorax (chest x-ray is diagnostic).

Management : Admit to hospital (1) if signs of severe asthma is present, (2) if the patient lives alone or is bed bound, (3) if he is no longer getting benefit from inhalers (Salbutamol inhaler up to 2 puffs/4h and beclomethasone inhaler up to 20 puffs/24 h). In addition to inhalers oral theophyllines are useful (slow release aminophylline 225 mg/12 hour or to produce a blood level of 10-15 mg/ml. Levels > 20 mg/ml may be toxic). Aminophylline suppositories are also useful (50 mg, 100 mg, 150 mg, 180 mg and 360 mg strengths. Dose example, 360 mg/120 h. pr). If these measures fail and IV therapy is not indicated maintain on oral prednosalone (ex. 4.5 mg/24 hours) which is of proven value. Avoid precipitating factors, discourage smoking. Those whose prick test (skin test) is positive to house dustmite extract will often be disappointed by exposure reduction (vacuum cleaning beds) and hyponsensitisation, even if bronchial provocation tests are positive.

Allopathy View and Treatment of Acute Asthma

Acute asthmatic attack presents with cyanosis, pulsus paradoxus, unable to speak, tachy or broadycardia, absent breath sounds (very severe asthma). Investigations include chest x-ray, arterial blood gases, peak expiratory growth rates.

An atmosphere of calm helps cure the patient. If severe, treat, otherwise, first investigate.

Use Salbutamol by nebulizer (0.5 to 1 ml in 2 ml 0.9% saline/ 4 hours) and if not better proceed as for severe.

Severe Immediate Therapy

a) Sit-up.

b) Give oxygen in high doses.

c) Hydrocortisone 200 mg bolus IV.

d) Aminophylline 250 mg IV (up to 5 mg/kg) IV as above.

e) Salbutamol nebulised as above, or 500 mg sc.

f) Check arterial blood gases, monitor pulsus paradoxus.

g) Arrange chest x-ray.

Severe Continuing Therapy

1) Continue giving oxygen.
2) Salbutamol nebulised as above, every 4 hours.
3) Aminophylline 1 mg/kg.
4) Cortisone 200 mg/6 hours IV.
5) IV Fluids : dextrose-saline 4l/24 hours to maintain urinary output.
6) Antibiotics + physiotherapy if there is chest infection.

Reassesment : If blood gas or pulsus paradoxus deteriorates consider ventilation (also if patient is exhausted or has cardiac arrest).

If blood gas improves after day one:

1) Stop hydrocortisone. Start prednisolone 40 mg/24 hr. Tail off after 1-2 weeks.
2) Stop aminophylline.
3) Cut down nebulised salbutamol. Switch to simple inhaler.

Allopathy has its own way of dealing with emergency states and certain parameters are followed as an index to treat. It will be interesting to compare with other systems mentioned below. Their approach and treatment are different.

Unani System of Medicine

Next to allopathy, let us consider the unani system about asthma. The unani system of medicine owes its origin to Hippocrates who laid the foundation for it in Greece between 460 and 377 BC. Abu Ali Sina, popularly known as Avicenna, too contributed significantly. It was later developed into an elaborate medical system by Arabs. Avicennas book *Al-Quandon* remained a reference book to unani doctors for many years. The unani system travelled through central Asia imbibing various traditional concepts of medicine and reached India around the 10th century AD.

Initially neglected, it slowly took firm root and flourished along with other Indian systems of medicine despite setbacks. An added impetus was given to it in the 1920's when the famous unani doctor, Masi Ul Mulk Hakim Ajmal Khan, engaged an eminent chemist, Dr. Salimuzzaman Siddhiqui, then with the Ayurvedic and Unani Tibbia College in Delhi to initiate research in unani medicine. Dr. Siddhiqui's subsequent discovery of the medicinal properties of Asrol (Chota Chand or Pagal Bhooti) led to the establishment of its efficacy in curing hypertension, insanity, schizophrenia, hysteria, insomnia and other psychosomatic conditions. This brought widespread recognition to the unani form of medicine from national and international medical circles.

In 1969, the government set up an autonomous institution, the Central Council for Research in Unani Medicine (CCRUM) for conducting research and disseminating knowledge in unani medicine. In 1978, CCRUM was split into four separate councils, one each for ayurveda and siddha, unani medicine, homeopathy, and yoga and natural cure.

The Unani Council has an ongoing programme of surveying the medicinal plants in the country. The work is being carried out at the councils Central Research Institute of Unani Medicine at Hyderabad, Andhra Pradesh, Central Herb Garden and Museum in Lucknow, and the Regional Research Institutes of Unani at Srinagar, Jammu and Kashmir, Aligarh, Uttar Pradesh, Bhadrak, Orissa and Chennai, Tamil Nadu. The survey has so far collected 35,000 plant species of which 23,000 have been provisionally identified. Experimental cultivation of a few unani herbs and shrubs to study their properties is also going on at the councils centres at Aligarh, Lucknow, Chennai, Srinagar. Considerable progress has been achieved in the cultivation of the some important plants such as *khatmi* (Althae officinalis), *aatrilal* (Ammi majus), *asal-us-soos* (Glycryrrhiza glabra) and others.

The Unani Medicine Council is engaged in establishing the efficacy of various unani drug formulations. It is conducting clinical trials on some endemic diseases such as filariasis, acute hepatitis, malaria, diabetes mellitus, asthma, renal calculi, amoebic dysentery, gastric ulcers, etc. The manufacture of unani drugs has been regularised through the Drugs and Cosmetics Act of 1940. The pharmocopeial standards for single and compound drug formulations have also been finalised. There exists a permanent unani pharmocopeia committee under the ministry of health and family welfare which consists of experts in unani medicine, chemists, botanists and pharmocologists. Today there are 22 undergraduate and two postgraduate colleges involved in teaching unani medicine. There are more than 100 unani hospitals and 1,000 dispensaries spread out in 16 states in the country. It now forms an integral part of our national health care delivery system.

Fundamental Concepts

Unani medicine takes a holistic view and treats the patient in relation to the environment in contrast to the allopathic system which views the patient as a biological organism that is under threat from other agents. Diet is given great importance in unani. It recommends abstinence from non-vegetarian food and lays stress on green vegetables and fruits. Regular, moderate exercises and proper rest to the body are also essential requirements to keep the muscles in good tone. Unani medicine is based on the Hippocratic theory, that a perfect balance of *arkan* (elements), *akhlat* (humours) and *mizaj* (temperament) helps in keeping the body healthy. Every individual is said to had an inherent power to self-preservation called the *Quwat-e-Modabira*. The Unani system of medicine is based on the humoral theory postulated by Hippocrates in his book *Tabeatal Insan* (Human Nature). The theory presupposes the presence of four humours in the human body :

1) Dum (blood)
2) Balgham (phlegm)
3) Safra (yellow bile)
4) Saoda (black bile)

Dum comprises all red fluids of the body while all colourless fluids are classified under *balgham*. Similarly yellow fluids are *safra* and black fluids are *saoda*. The *mizaj* (behavioural pattern) of a person is expressed by the preponderance of a particular humour. Unani medicine assigns the following four temperaments:

1) *Damvi* (sanguine or plethoric)
2) *Safravi* (choleric or bilious)
3) *Balghami* (cold or phlegmatic)

4) *Saodvi* (melancholic)

A distinctive feature of unani medicine is the emphasis on diagnosing disorders primarily through the *nabi* (pulse). The doctors also resort to pathological tests on *baul* (urine) and *baraz* (stools). The examination of the urine and stool is considered important, and the findings are examined in conjunction with the readings made through the pulse examination. With the advent of modern methods of chemical analysis and imaging these have been readily accepted to help in better diagnosis of disorders. Ibn-al-Nafees; an ancient physician, in his book *Al-al-Din-Qarshi* stated the fundamental principles of pulse examination including the rhythmical contraction (systole) and expansion (diastole) of the heart which could be felt through the pulse.

A Unani doctor looks for the following information while examining the pulse :

1) *Miqdar* (volume)
2) *Kafiyathal* (tension)
3) *Qiwamal alah* (condition of the blood vessels)
4) *Miqdar mafil shiryan* (blood volume)
5) *Zamana-al-harqat* (duration and rate of the movement)
6) *Zamana al sukoon* (duration of rest)
7) *Malmas* (tactus)
8) *Istawa-e-kaifyath* (rhythm)
9) *Nizam and adam nizam* (rest and irregularity)
10) *Wazn* (equilibrium)

Treatment in the unani system of medicine is done mainly through diet control for simple diseases in the initial stages followed by the administration of a single drug failing which compound preparations may be administered. Every single drug is divided into categories from I to IV according to their potency and efficacy.

The various treatment therapies available under the unani system are therapies such as :

1) *Ilaj bit-tad beer* (regimental therapy)

2) *Ilaj bil—ghiya* (dietotherapy)

3) *Ilajbiddawa* (pharmocotherapy)

4) *Jawahat* (surgery).

The regimental therapy includes methods such as venesection, cupping, diaphoresis, diuresis, turkish bath, massage, metastasis, cauterisation, purging, emesis, exercise, leaching and many more.

The dietotherapy aims at treating certain ailments by controlling the intake of food and regulating the quality of the food. In pharmocotherapy the doctors use naturally occurring drugs, mostly herbal though drugs of animal origin are also used. The advantage with the natural drugs are that most of them do not have any harmful side effects unlike the powerful allopathic drugs.

Bronchial Asthma/(Zeeaun-Nafs)

Asthma, referred to as *Zeeaun-nafs* in unani medicine, is characterised by paroxysms of breathlessness which is accompanied by wheezing as a result of the narrowing of the airways or accumulation of viscids secretions. Unani specialists attribute this disease to the disorder with the *balgham* (phlegm). Avicenna described it as a phlegmatic chronic disorder which occurs with great frequency. It may be aggravated by internal or external factors. A person may be afflicted at any age and both the sexes are equally affected. In the initial stage, the person can feel the congestion building up in his chest. During the attack the patient feels breathless. The attack which could be aggravated by external factors like pollen dust, grass, feather, dust, smoke and tobacco among other things, may last two to three hours. It could also be triggered by psychological factors and indigestion.

Prevention and Treatment

1) Five ml of ginger juice taken before sleep helps in preventing an attack.

2) One teaspoonful of turmeric powder mixed with a glass of milk keeps the phlegm away and prevents the attack.

3) Fifty gms ajwain seeds are to be mixed with a little ginger and 5 gms taken twice daily.

4) *Abhal* (juniper berry) 10 gms
Maghz Amaltas (Indian laburnum) 10 gms
Zanjabeel (ginger) 5 gms
mix and take 1 gm daily.

Ayurveda

Ayurveda is a comprehensive system of health care, and its many elements work together for specific illnesses. Ayurveda and its relation to Indian philosophy is derived from the *Vedas*, the divine Hindu books of knowledge. The aim of ayurveda is not only healing of the sick, but the prevention of illness and the preservation of life. In that way it comprises a noble system of living that it ayurveda the most complete system of medicine and health care we know today. Some of the elements of ayurvedic medicine include :

a) Detoxification by *pancha karma*
b) Diet
c) Yoga
d) Herbal medication
e) Medication and prayer.

The basic ayurvedic belief is that everything within the universe including ourselves is composed of five elements called *Panchamahabhutas* and *Tridoshas*. By correcting the balance of the *tridoshas* within ourselves and in relation to the world around us, we will promote health at all levels. Ayurvedic treatment is tailored to the individual. There is no other treatment that works for an ailment in every person. The combination of the *doshas* that make up one person might lead to optimum health for them. In another person that balance of *doshas* may cause an illness.

In ayurvedic medicine, every person must be treated individually. The skill of the practitioner lies in assessing each individual's constitution, diagnosing the causes of any imbalance, identifying the constitutional type and where the balance of *doshas* lie, and deciding upon the best possible treatment. Ayurveda is aimed at treating the mind, body and spirit. *Vata-pita-kapha* are the *tridoshas*. Each individual's constitution is controlled by all three doshas to different degrees, but usually one or possibly two dominant *doshas* decide the constitution. *Doshas* determine the characteristics of our constitution and the type of illnesses to which we are most likely to succumb. Good health reigns when all three *doshas* work in balance. The *three doshas* or the bioenergetic forces govern our health and determine our *prakriti* (physical constitution). Ayurveda is a holistic system of health care that teaches us to balance these energies in order to achieve optimum health and well being and to preserve life. The emphasis on maintaining good health or swasthvartta is crucial in ayurveda. The daily routine or dinacharya and the seasonal regimen or ritucharya are designed to keep us healthy. In *dinacharya* diet, physical exercise, personal hygiene and mental health are all important. The three *doshas* have different functions:

Pittas functions are : Vision, digestion, heat production, imparting colour to body, hunger, thirst appetite, softness and suppleness of the body and all intellectual functions.

Kapha functions : Maintaining illness of body and organs,

	maintaining general stability of body, providing strength, patience, virility, promoting smooth working of joints, forebearance, courage, generosity
Functions of *vata* are :	Imparting motion to body (praspandanam), conducting impulses from respective sense organs (*udvahanam*), separating egesta which is a waste from ingested food (*virek*), retaining and evacuating urine and semen (*dharanam*).

Vata consists of predominance of *vayu* and *akasha* (air and space).

Pitta consists of *tejas* and *jala* (fire and water).

Kapha is formed by *jala* and *prithvi* (water and earth).

When the three *doshas* are in balance and in normal state, they bring about good health, growth, strength, happiness, mental stability and complexion. When the three *doshas* are unbalanced or in an abnormal state, they cause various diseases.

Unbalanced *vata* causes	→	Rheumatism, arthritis, stomach pain, constipation, circulatory problems, etc.
Unbalanced *pitta* causes	→	Acidity, skin eruptions, anger, hysteria.
Unbalanced *kapha* causes	→	Obesity, nausea, bronchitis, asthma, heaviness in head, loss of memory.

Abnormal *vata* causes 80 types of disease.

Abnormal *pitta* cases 40 types of diseases.

Abnormal *kapha* cases 20 types of diseases.

Ayurveda has cures for most, if not all, chronic ailments. There are a number of cases where ayurvedic medicine cannot have immediate effect and the patient can develop serious complications as in acute infections and illnesses, myocardial infarction, emergency surgery cases.

A number of ayurvedic medicines and oils are used by Western trained physicians in India as adjuncts to Western medicine. Ayurveda is useful in the treatment of many conditions like constipation, eczema, colds, anxiety, high BP, allergies, sinusitis, back pain, insomnia, headaches, paralysis, etc.

Daily routines included in the ayurvedic concept of healthy living are (1) early rising, (2) cleanliness, (3) exercise (*kaphaja* persons can perform heavy exercise; *pittika* persons should do exercises in moderation; *vata* people can take up yoga and not aerobic exercise), (4) satisfying natural urges, mental and moral discipline. Diets are prescribed for rainy season, fall, winter, spring and summer separately.

Diagnosis in Ayurveda

As we have studied, the imbalance of the *doshas* that govern physical and mental health is responsible for diseases. Imbalance has three causes:

i) Abnormal or unhealthy contact of sense organs with certain objects. This is called *Asatmyendriyartha samyoga.*

ii) Errors in judgement (*Prajnaparadha*)

iii) The influence of time and the season (*Parinama*).

Diagnostic techniques in ayurvedic include:

1) Examination of the patient : this includes :

a) Assessment of the cause of disease or *nidana*

b) Early signs and symptoms or *purvaroopa*

c) Main signs and symptoms or *roopa*

d) Exploratory therapy or *upasaya*

e) The production of disease or *samprapti*

2) Clinical examination of the patient.

Textual knowledge (*aptopadesa*)

Direct perception (*pratyaksha*) } These three are important

Inference (*anumana*) } for clinical examination

Examination (*Astavidha pariksha*).

Examination of the patients may be tenfold.

Examination (*dashvidha pariksha*) eightfold

The tenfold fold examination involves :

1) Body constitution (*prakriti*)
2) Pathological state (*vikriti*)
3) Tissue vitality (*sara*)
4) Physical build (*sambanana*)
5) Body measurement (*pramana*)
6) Adaptability (*satmya*)
7) Psychic constitution (*sattva*)
8) Digestive capacity (*ahara shakti*)
9) Capacity of exercise (*vyanama shakti*)
10) Age (*vaya*)

The eightfold examination includes :

1) Examination of pulse (*nadi pariksha*)
2) Examination of tongue (*jivha pariksha*)
3) Examination of voice (*sabda parikha*)
4) Examination of skin (*sparsha pariksha*)
5) Examination of the eye (*drka pariksha*)
6) Examination of general appearance (*akrti pariksha*)
7) Examination of urine (*mutra pariksha*)
8) Examination of stool (*mala pariksha*)

Classification of Diseases in Ayurveda

1) Curable or incurable
2) Mild or severe
3) Endogenous and exogenous
4) Medical or surgical

Classification can also be done on the basis of :

1) predominant *dosha* involved
2) site of body involved
3) main symptoms
4) structure of body
5) change of colour of body
6) the origin.

Treatment in Ayurveda

Treatment includes :

1) Drugs (*aushadha*)
2) Diet (*anna*)
3) Practices (*vihara*)

The four pillars of treatment are:

Physician, medicament, attendant, patient.

The four forms of treatment are :

1) Medicine or drug therapy
2) *Panchakarma* (the five systems of treatment)
3) Dietary regime
4) Regulation of lifestyle.

Ayurveda works in two fundamental ways < Prevention / Cure

The *preventive aspect* of ayurvedic medicine has three parts, namely, (1) personal hygiene (2) rejuvenation and virilification and (3) yoga.

1) Personal hygiene is called *svasthavarta*. This also includes *sadachara* or appropriate behaviour.
2) Rejuvenation (*rasayana* and *vajikarana*)
3) Virilification (*vajikarana*)

Yoga keeps the body and mind in excellent condition.

The *curative aspect* of ayurvedic medicine has three parts again:

1) Internal medicine (*antati parimaijana*)—uses enema, purgation, etc.
2) External medicine (*vahir parimaijana*)—uses massage, pastes, powders, oblations.
3) Surgical treatment (*shastra pranidhana*) this is very rare today except for fistula.

Ayurveda describes 10 proper occasions to take medicine.

Abpukta	—	on empty stomach
Pragbhukta	—	before a meal
Adhobhukta	—	after a meal
Antarabhukta	—	between meals
Madhyabhukta	—	in the course of a meal
Sabhukta	—	mixed with the meal
Samudga	—	given at the beginning and end of the meal
Muhurmuhu	—	repeatedly
Grass	—	with every morsel of food

Grasanter — with each alternate morsel of food.

There are three types of massage and 32 surgical manoeuvres which are special to ayurveda but they will not be elaborated here. Ayurvedic treatment also includes psychotherapy and spiritual therapy. This is known as *Satwavajaya.*

Pankaja-Kasturi, an ayurvedic medicinal preparation, has been very effective in breathlessness caused by certain conditions. It has a lot of ingredients which make breathing easy.

The preparation is available as a semisolid *Lehiam* (paste), syrup and also as sugar-free preparation for diabetics. This Ayurvedic preparation contains:

1) Piper tongum
2) Piper nigrum
3) Zinzibar officinalis.
4) Elettaria cardamom
5) Cinnamum cassia
6) Withania somnisera
7) Tamarindus indica
8) Cuminum cyminum
9) Aegle marmelos
10) Adhatoda vasica
11) Terminalia chebula
12) Terminalia blerica
13) Tragia inbolucrata
14) Rubia cordifolia along with sugar candy in the standard form.

As we see, it has ingredients like ginger, pepper, etc.

Indications for use are in conditions of breathlessness, as in tonsillitis, allergic bronchitis, eosonophilia, cough and for general health.

This preparation is sold in all allopathy medical stores and is very popular in Tamil Nadu.

Panchakarma is '5' purification therapies used in ayurveda to treat certain conditions. They are detoxification procedures aimed more at prevention measures rather than cure.

Yoga and Spiritual Remedies

Yoga is a science as well as a method of achieving spiritual harmony through the control of mind and body. The *asanas* (yogic postures) and *pranayama* (breath control) are practices that not only help us to acquire perfect health, but also develop a calm and serene mind. Yoga is an essential part of ayurveda. Its meaning comes from a Sanskrit word which indicates the total integration of the individual soul with the Supreme or Divine Soul to obtain relief from pain and suffering.

Prayers, *mantras*, remedial rituals are an essential part of ayurveda, particularly for chronic serious ailments. The diseases are the product of individual *karma* ('doing'). The only way to transcend the negative *karma* is through good actions and the invocation of divine help through *mantras* and prayer. A good ayurvedic physician will be able to guide a person regarding this aspect.

Ayurveda and Asthma

Asthma in ayurveda comes under the category of respiratory diseases. One of the three *doshas* or a combination of these *doshas* can trigger asthma. In many cases, it is also a hereditary factor. In ayurveda mainly education is imparted to the patient. Ayurveda can do nothing for acute asthma. The patient is then referred to an allopath. The individual has a greater role to play than the physician because a lot of importance to his food habits is given and there is a great amount of importance given also to external atmosphere.

The patient has to be aware of how to manage himself in certain weather conditions and the diet he has to follow under the circumstances. The person is more important than the doctor. The more cooperative the patient is, the more effective is the result. The patient should have faith in the medicine and the doctor. Ayurveda has its limitations in the sense that it is 'more preventive'. Once the attack sets in, very little can be done. The person has to be referred to a system which can do better than ayurveda. Also if the patient is very old treating becomes a problem. In ayurveda, asthma is dealt more on preventive aspects as mentioned earlier.

Three categories of treatment are used:

Ahara — food habits
- what to eat
- when to eat
- how to eat
- in what combination

Vihara — deals with external atmosphere

If the above two cannot prevent the disease, *aushadha* or medicine is resorted to *Adosha (Adhatoda Vasica Nees),* an evergreen shrub seen through out the plains of India, commonly found near habitations, has lance-shaped leaves. The leaves and roots are used medicinally. They contain an alkaloid vasicine. In the ayurvedic system of medicine, it comes under *Kasaghna Gana* (anti tussive). It is an expectorant, antispasmodic, tonic and blood purifier. *Adosha* is used in treatment of many ailments of respiratory tract including asthma. One tablespoon juice of leaves with equal quantity of honey thrice daily is very useful in cough. This mixture is used in asthma.

Siddha and homoeopathy also have their methods of curing/ preventing asthma.

Siddha

'Pulse' is used to the rhythmic waves which are of three kinds: *vatam* (anabolic force), *kapam* (catabolic force) and *pittam* (metabolic force). *Nadi* reading is main in the siddha system. Food and lifestyle changes are prescribed in this system. Though this system uses metals as medicine (in converting the metals into medicine, toxic contents are eliminated by oxidising the metals with juices of numerous plants), it is done in extreme stages of disease only. For asthma normally metallic medicines are not given. The siddha system of medicine has been a very ancient system of medicine in India passed on through generations by siddhars or men who had miraculous healing powers.

Homoeopathy

The basis of homeopathy medicine system is a philosophy called "Law of Similars", otherwise known as "Like Cures like". This means that a substance that produces symptoms in a healthy person can cure a person suffering from the same symptoms. For example, if eating a certain herb causes people to cough that same herb is used to treat a sick person whose main symptom is cough. The goal is to stimulate the immune system so that the body heals itself. Homoeopathy originated 200 years ago in protest against harsh medical practices of the day such as blood letting, purging, etc. Homoeopathic medications are highly diluted versions of plant, herb, animal extracts. Recently, a British medical journal surveyed various homeopathic studies and concluded certain remedies might be effective especially for seasonal allergies. Homeopathy cannot treat acute attacks of asthma. Preventive aspects of asthma can be tackled using homoeopathy. Certain critics say that (1) if you take homeopathy drug, you run the risk of not getting treatment for serious medical conditions. (2) Homoeopathic drugs should be avoided in life-threatening or chronic illnesses. (3) Many homoeopathic extracts are preserved in alcohol and this alcohol (like that in mouth washes) may increase the risk of oral cancer.

Yoga

Yoga forms an important part in the treatment regime of ayurveda. When patients come with asthma to yoga therapists, they are often in a state of fear and anxiety. They wonder whether there is any hope at all for them. In chronic illness, the entire person becomes ill, not just the physical body or a particular part of the body. Therefore, first the yoga therapist builds a rapport with the patient before introducing yoga training. The teacher of yoga has to instil confidence in the person by giving some examples. The patient has to relax. Then the posture is improved. It is made sure that the person can contract the stomach to breathe out. The abdomen region is sometimes tense in such cases.

People who come to yoga teachers are often under treatment with various medicines. The yoga teacher tells them that they have a lot of potential within them and the greater the responsibility the patient takes the sooner they will become better. A patient gets better if he or she has the inclination and the responsibility. Any limitations in the system are the limitations of the person. We have already discussed yogic exercises in asthma, hence we will just mention two things here:

1) *Sarvanga Asana* (the shoulder stand posture) and its variation *Dvipadapitham* bring relief to asthmatic patients. They remove respiratory defects in the lungs through internal activation, and all parts of the body are exercised, energised and activated.

2) *Chakravakasana* is also a very valuable *asana* for asthmatics.

We have already discussed about *pranayama* and its role in asthma. This control of breathing achieved by one particular *pranayama* (*kapalabhati*), brings relief in asthmatics. In yoga, more than the actual intervention it is the quality of the person, who is providing the intervention that is paramount. The quality of yoga healer is very important. In ayurveda also the quality of the healer is an important aspect in healing.

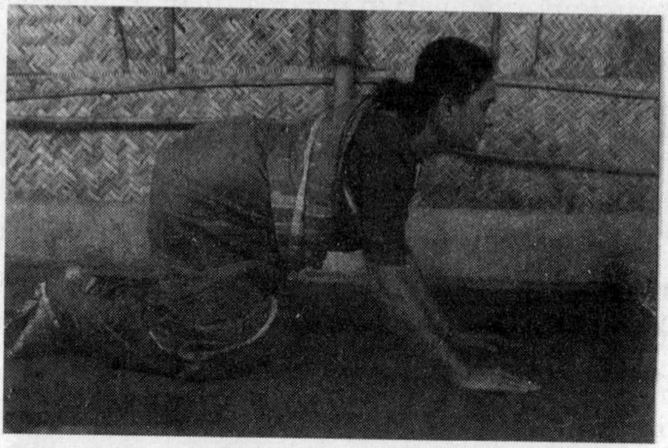

Chakravakasana

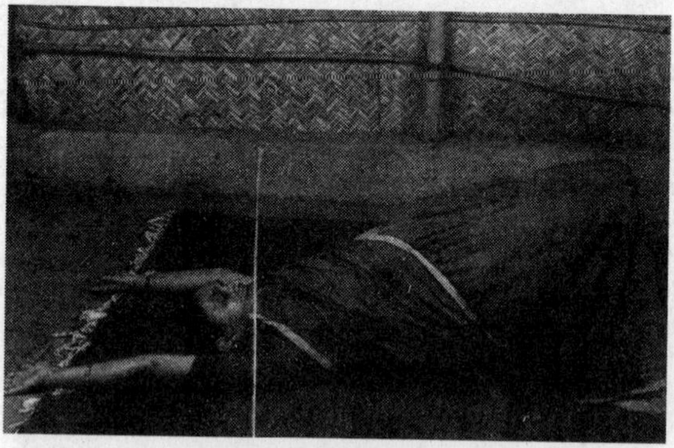

Dvipadapitham

Yoga, 'the science of human development', also has some solutions for asthma. This being a part of ayurveda (which we have already discussed in detail) needs no more detailed explanations.

Pranic Healing

This is a no-touch, no-drug therapeutic method of holistic healing. The term *pranic* originates from the Sanskrit word 'Prana' which means vital energy or life force. It is this energy that helps to keep our body alive and healthy. There are three major sources of *prana,* namely, solar *prana*, air *prana*, ground *prana.* Pranic healing also has been called by many other names like *Medical ki* or energy healing, psychic healing, vitalic healing, faith healing, charismatic healing. Originating from the Indian subcontinent, it has come back to us in its modern version.

Pranic healing is based on the overall structure of the human body. Man's physical body is composed of two parts (1) the visible physical body (2) the invisible energy body, aura or the bioplasmic body is the name given to this body. The energy body has fine bioplasmic channels or meridians or *nadis*. It is through this channels that the vital energy force called *ki* or bioplasmic matter flows and is distributed all over our body. Sickness in one physical body is accompanied by the excess *prana* or energy in localised areas of our body. This is called *Pranic Congestion*. Sometimes meridians are blocked leading to *Pranic Depletion*. These conditions are treated by a process of cleansing and energising using the healer himself as a medium to channel healing energy of divine origin. Our invisible energy body has "whirling energy centres" or "chakras". These are affected in disease. In *pranic* healing (1) in areas of congestion, the diseased energy is removed from the affected areas (2) water is used to absorb the negative energy, (3) in areas of *pranic* depletion cleansing and energising are applied to the affected area with the emphasis being on energising, (4) the healer projects the healing *prana* to the affected area. Anybody can learn and practise *pranic* healing. *Pranic* healing can heal many physical, mental and emotional ailments by 'No Touch-No Drug' therapy. There is also *pranic self healing* and distant healing techniques.

The cause for asthma can be external but there is an internal cause also. The internal cause is divided into two: one is the emotional cause. If a person does not express the full potential that he is born with, then he will slowly start feeling suffocated. All diseases start with the mind, then it slowly becomes physical. There is another internal cause known as *karmic* reason. It implies that as you sow, you will reap. Some *pranic* healing gurus give examples of some small children who caught hold of a few kittens, put them in a bag and watched them choke to death. These children then of course suffered from asthma. The same would apply to those who put crabs into boiling water and watch them die. In asthma, the person experiences what is called a choking reaction. Therefore, if the cause is emotional, then it will physicalise itself in the form of choking. Asthma is the inability to breathe in or breathe out. In *pranic* healing, both the 'energy body' and the 'physical body' are treated because for true healing to take place both these entities need normalising. If the disease is due to physical reasons, like pollens, house dust or food allergy, then dealing with asthma is easy. The patient sits in a receptive pose and the healer does the healing. The patient plays a role in the sense that he avoids whatever is causing the asthma till the energy body is strong enough and it physicialises on the physical body. When the cause is emotional, the healing is done on the energy body. The patient is advised not to pity himself. The emotion of self-pity affects the back heart *chakra* which controls the lungs. The patients are asked to meditate and stay happy. This way the patient is involved in his own healing. A good healer is also a very important factor in *pranic* healing. *Pranic* healing is impossible without the patient's cooperation.

Magneto Therapy

What does magneto therapy have for asthma ? Magneto therapy is a natural treatment and does not involve drugs. This external application can go with any other system of treatment or medicines. It is a harmless, safe, simple, cheap and economical treatment at home. It is a recognised science in various countries like USA, Russia, Japan, Italy, France, Australia, etc. It has been conclusively proved that chronic diseases which are otherwise incurable with the conventional systems of medicine readily respond to magneto therapy.

1) *The Effect of North Pole Magnet*: The North Pole gives cooling effect and cures boils, eczema, itching, obesity and arrests growth of bacteria and cancer. It is to be applied on the right, front, outerside, upperside of the affected parts of the body.

2) *The Effect of South Pole Magnet*: The South Pole provides heat, energy, strength, removes stiffness, pains, swellings, and improves blood circulations. It is to be used on the left side, back, inside and under affected parts of the body.

High Power Magnet

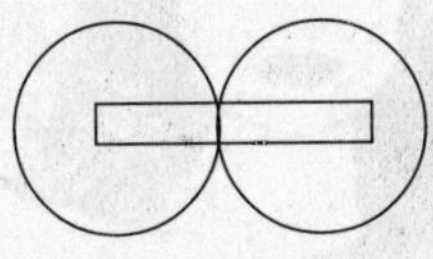

Fig. 9.1 : High Power Magnet

Use the North Pole under the right hand palm and the South Pole under the left hand palm. It is for treatment of ailments of the upper side of the body as pains, asthma, heart troubles, arthritis, paralysis of legs. Place the North Pole under the sole of the right foot and South Pole under the sole of the left foot. It can be used to make magnetised water and oil.

Lower power magnets are used on the nose, eyes, ears, and throat for treating infants.

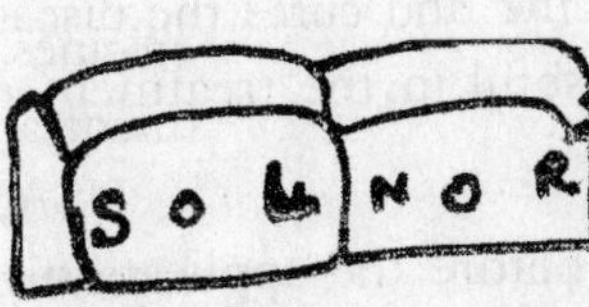

Fig. 9.2 : Low Power Magnets

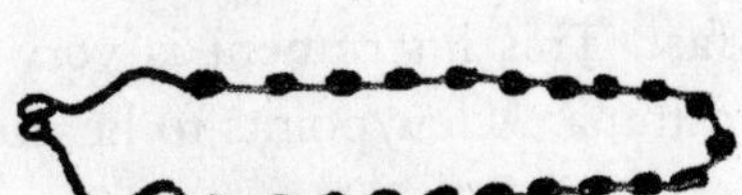

Fig. 9.3 : Asthma Chain

Asthma Chain

The asthma chain can be worn throughout the day and night (except while taking bath) for relief in ailments of chest, namely, asthma, bronchitis, inflammation, pains, cold, etc.

Headache Belt

The headache belt can be tied around the forehead for 30 minutes once or twice a day for the complaints of brain, headache, *migraine*, mental weakness, retardation, and insomnia.

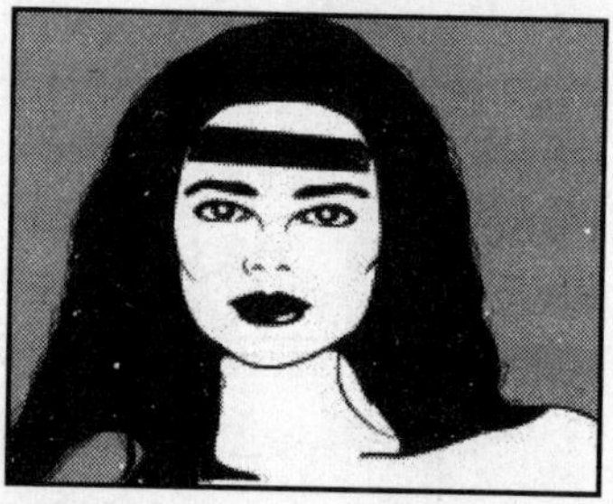

Fig. 9.4 : Headache Belt

You also have a health or BP watch for high/low blood pressures; obesity belt for diabetes, hernia, uterine diseases, etc. There is also a knee belt for arthritis, gout, knee swelling; magnetic spectacles for cataract, burning eyes, etc.

Electromagnetic Pulser

This instrument can be used in clinics and houses. The magnetic waves coming out of this instrument are useful in relieving pain, injuries, chest pain, neck pain, etc. It should be used only 10 minutes at a time. An electromagnetic pulser, when used along with permanent magnets, is more effective and cures the disease fast. This instrument is very much useful in the treatment of asthma. A few points to be noted are :

1) The watch should be removed before the application of magnets.

2) The patient should not take ice-creams or cold drinks for an hour after their application.

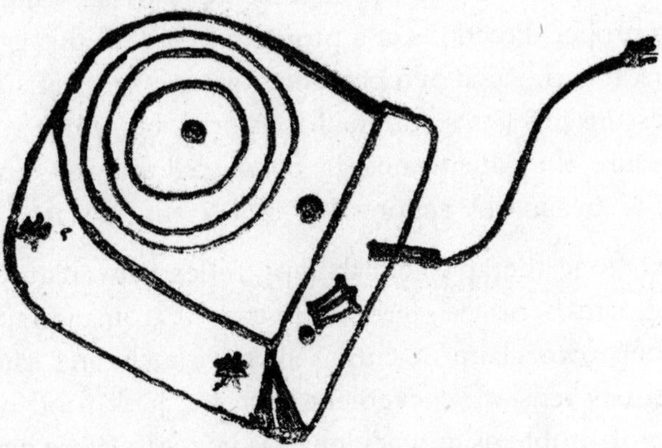

Fig. 9.5 : Electromagnet Pulser

3) Strong magnets should not be applied to pregnant ladies and during menses period, to the delicate organs like heart, brain, eyes.

4) They should also not take a bath for an hour after its use.

Former England Prime Minister, Margaret Thatcher, looked youthful and attractive after using magnetised water.

This often does not work in advanced stages of the disease. If the cause of the disease is physical, the chances are that the patient will be healed quickly, but not if the cause is emotional and if the patient is really anxious to get well. Success has been achieved in not many, but few cases; if it is *karmic*, then it takes time. Sometimes it is impossible.

Acupressure

Apply pressure with your fingertips for a minute or two on certain points so that a balance is created in the body energy flow and this cures the disease. It is a Chinese system which travelled to the USA and some European countries. Now it is also popular in

India. We all have energy flowing within us. This energy is created by the food we take and the lifestyle we lead. This energy has to flow in proper directions at a proper time and if this is disturbed, the person complains of a particular disease/problems ailing him. Acupressure too has solutions for asthma, but when resorting to acupressure, the patient must be convinced that the healer knows the art of healing by acupressure in a scientific way.

Reiki, zone therapy, gem therapy, reflexology, nature cure and cure by pyramids/magnets (has been discussed), aromatherapy all these have their own claim in curing allergies including asthma. The modern day tension, excitement, fast life, junk food brings in a number of problems in one's life. It is better to lead a happy active life by taking one of these alternative systems of healing, depending upon one's needs.

That Fishy Feeling

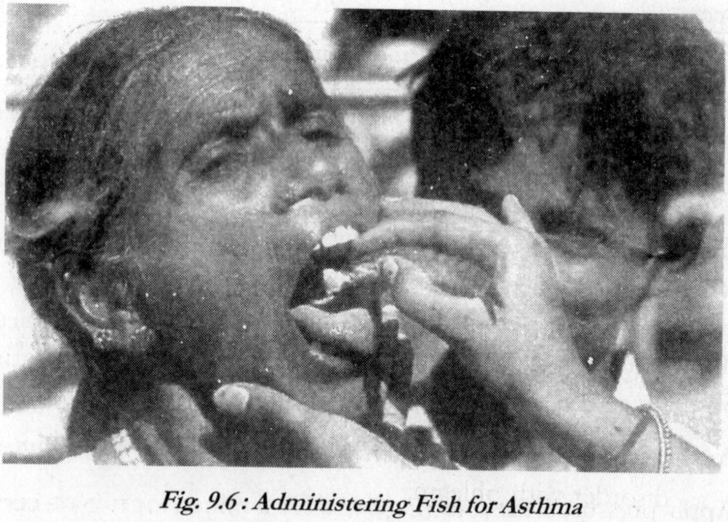

Fig. 9.6 : Administering Fish for Asthma

Sceptics routinely complain about an annual asthma cure event in Hyderabad but it only draws bigger crowds of hopefuls—'at least three lakhs every year'—for the one-day affair on a particular date well advertised before. The bizzare ritual involves a three year-in-a-row dose of a secret formula administered with a raw two-inch river fish called murrel. Each dose has to be followed by a 45-day diet which includes 26 items such as old rice and figs and precludes buffalo milk and chicken. Shivaram Gowd, a small time landlord (who offers this 'cure' with his four brothers), says, "We cannot explain this phenomenon, except that our family has been 'chosen' to perform this sacred duty." He claims it was passed down by a sadhu in 1845 who ordained that the dose must be administered on a day sacred to Telugus, on *Mrugasira Kartik*. The event draws people from outside the state. For the first time there was even a special train from Guwahati; usually coaches are added to Hyderabad bound trains. The Gowds prepare and pay for the formulation (50 kgs— Rs. 22,000), the police manage the crowd, volunteers provide the Rs. 2 fish at cost, water, shelter and help administer doses on assembly line fashion Worth it? Maybe, maybe not.

> Ajay Kabra from Madhya Pradesh complained to Gowd that he was not cured even after his three visits. Gowd did not bat an eyelid and said that he needed a double dose. Kabra dejectedly rejoined another, serpentine queue. "I am desperate," he griped, "I need a cure".

Summary

1. Allopathy offers preventive and curative solutions to asthma. Acute asthma can be managed with allopathy.
2. Unani offers certain simple home remedies (ginger, turmeric) for asthma. The specialists attribute asthma to disorder with phlegm.
3. Ayurveda cannot do anything for acute attacks. It offers preventive treatment. Medicines, diet and modifications in external environment are offered in the treatment package.

4. Yoga, often a part of Ayurveda treatment, cannot do anything for *acute* attacks, but helps in asthma prevention and treatment by *asanas* and *pranayama.*
5. *Pranic* healing treats energy body and physical body to get results. Patient's cooperation is very important in healing.
6. Magnetotherapy offers asthma chain and electromagnet pulser for the treatment of asthma.

10

ALLERGY : A READER-FRIENDLY SECTION

Allergy

This is a reader-friendly section answering many common queries on allergy in a very simple language and in easy-to- understand terms.

What is allergy ?

Allergy is a kind of an over-reaction by the body to a substance which causes most people little or no harm. Such substances are called allergens. The cells of the body identify them as harmful foreign substances and thus try to fight the invasion.

Who can develop an allergy?

One person out of four has a tendency to develop allergic reaction to some substance or another. The problem in allergic people is that their immune system reacts to apparently harmless substances such as food or pollen as if it were an unwanted invader.

Which parts of the body are affected by allergy?

1) Nose
2) Eyes
3) Lungs
4) Skin

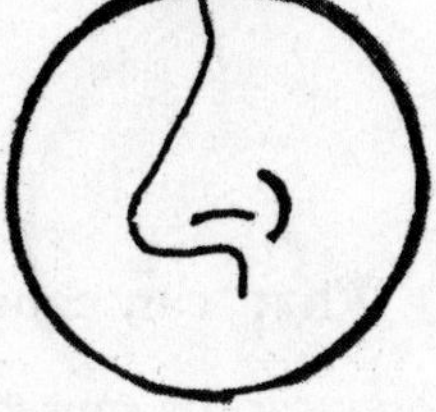

Fig. 10.1 : Nose

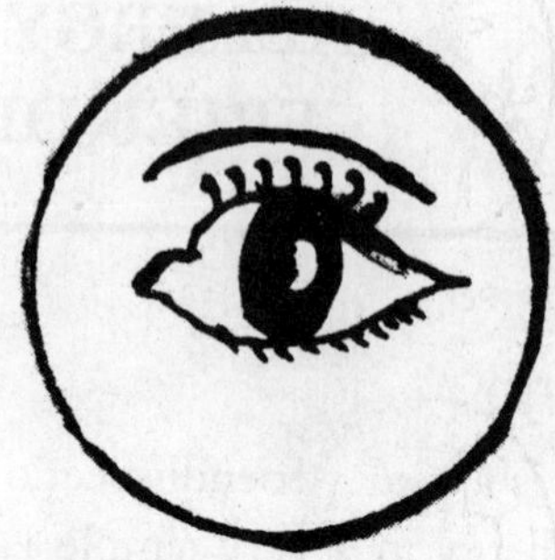

Fig. 10.2 : Eyes

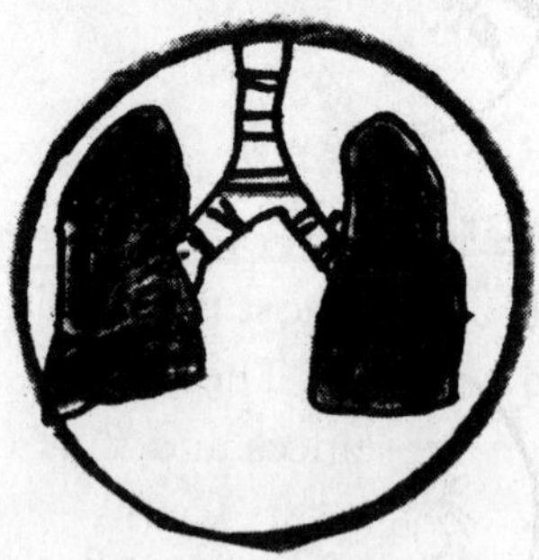

Fig. 10.3 : Lungs

Fig. 10.4 : Skin

What can cause allergy?

Allergy can be caused by just about anything. Although the list is endless, a few of the common allergens are mentioned:

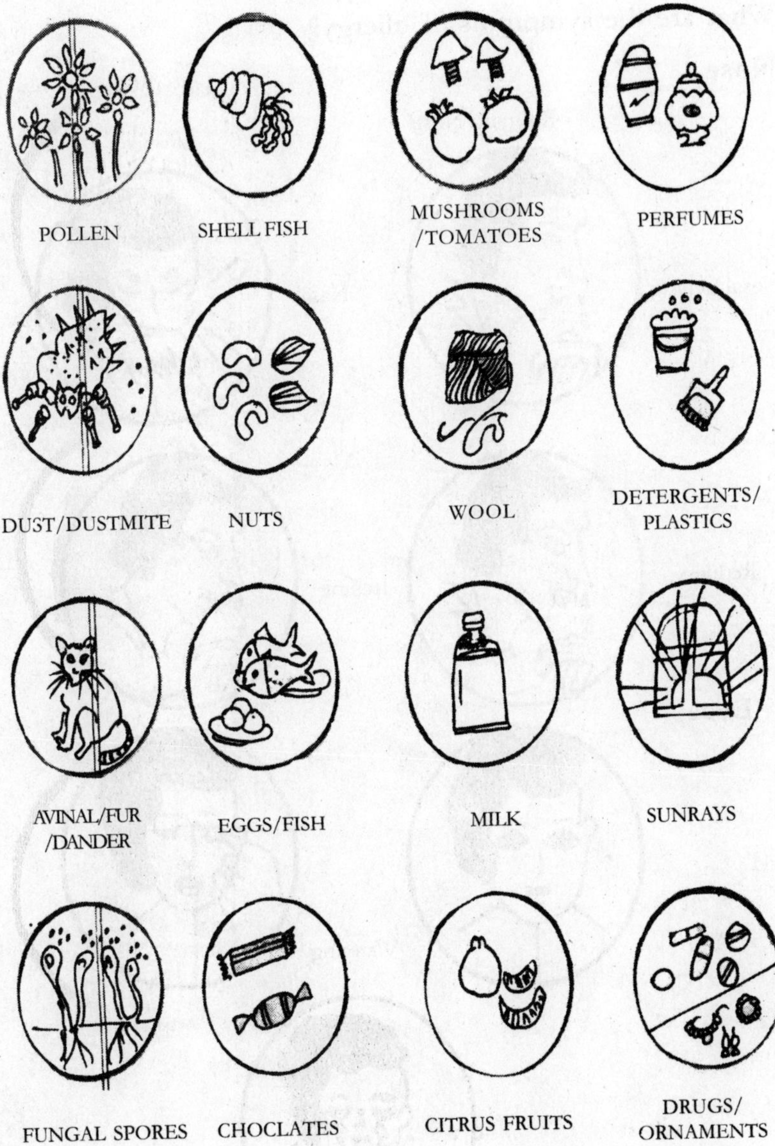
POLLEN
SHELL FISH
MUSHROOMS /TOMATOES
PERFUMES
DUST/DUSTMITE
NUTS
WOOL
DETERGENTS/ PLASTICS
AVINAL/FUR /DANDER
EGGS/FISH
MILK
SUNRAYS
FUNGAL SPORES
CHOCLATES
CITRUS FRUITS
DRUGS/ ORNAMENTS

Fig. 10.5 : Possible Causes of Allergy

What are the symptoms of allergy?

Nose

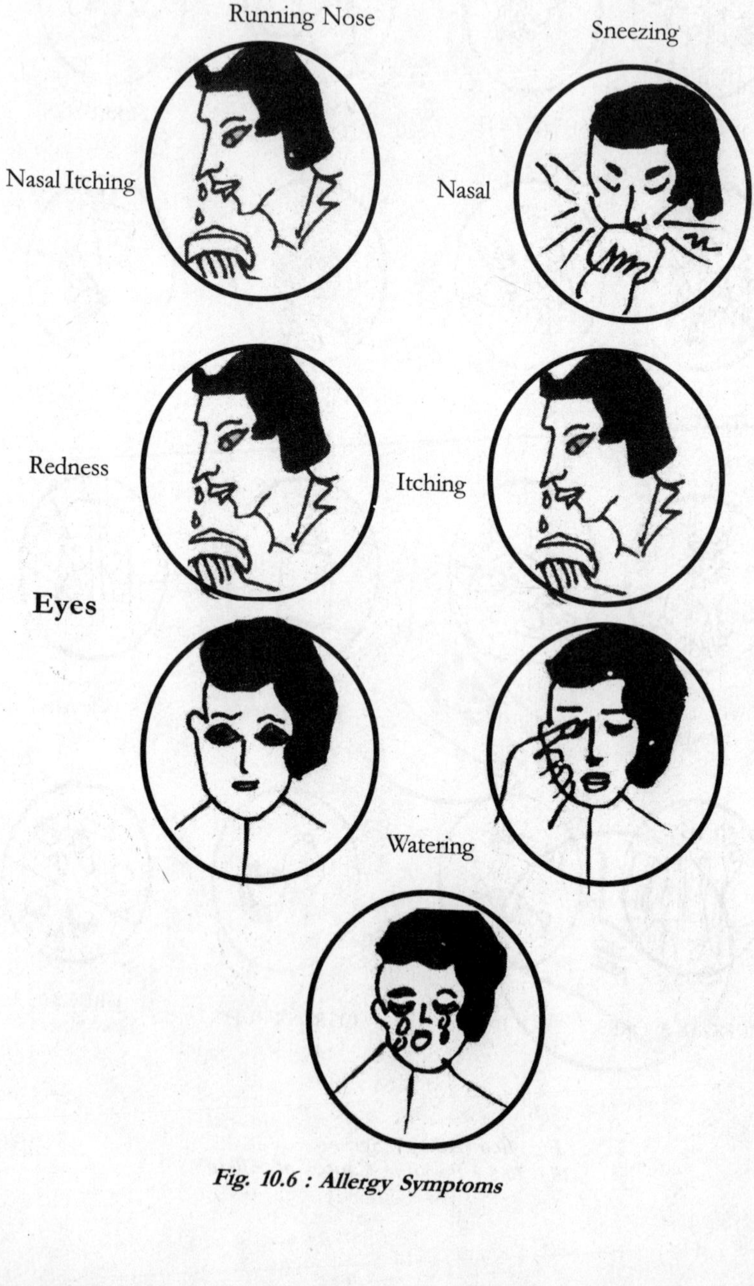

Fig. 10.6 : Allergy Symptoms

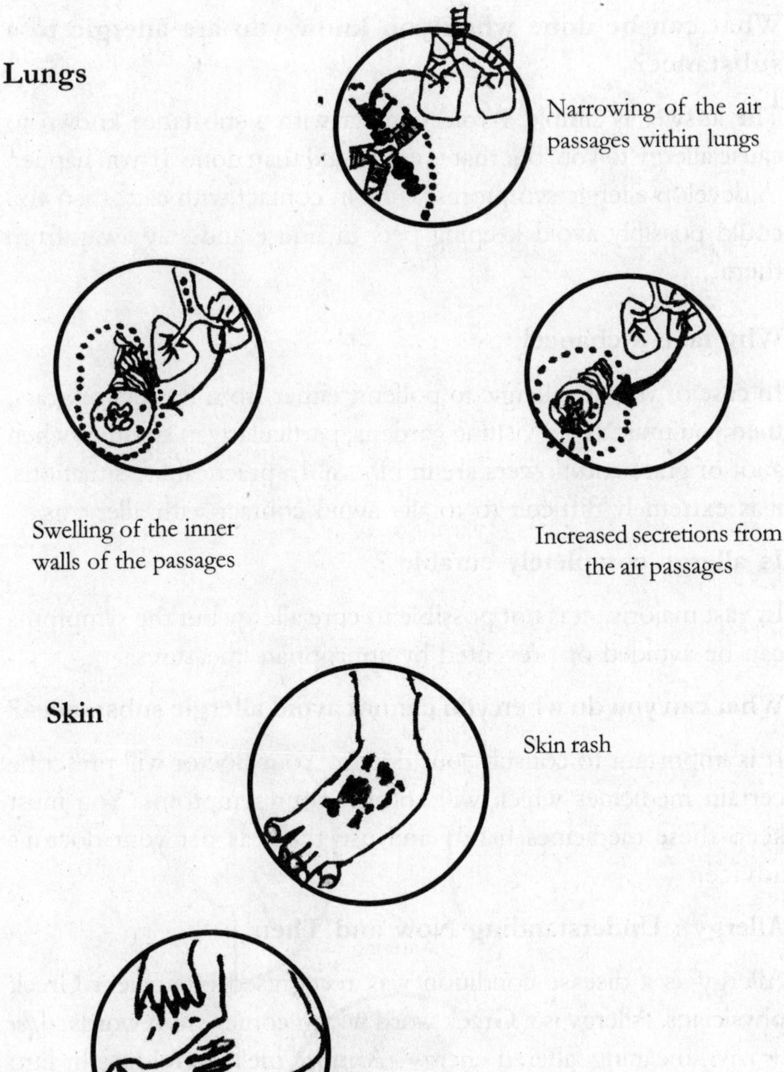

Fig. 10.6 **(*Allergy Symptoms*)**

What can be done when you know you are allergic to a substance?

The answer is simple. Avoid contact with a substance known to cause allergy to you, but that is easily said than done. If you happen to develop allergic symptoms while in contact with cats, then you could possibly avoid keeping pets in house and stay away from them.

Why take a chance!

In case of you are allergic to pollens, either from flowers or grass, then you must avoid visiting gardens, particularly in summer when a lot of grass and flowers are in bloom. In practical life situations, it is extremely difficult to totally avoid contact with allergens.

Is allergy completely curable ?

In vast majority, it is not possible to cure allergy but the symptoms can be avoided or prevented by appropriate measures.

What can you do when you cannot avoid allergic substances?

It is important to consult your doctor. Your doctor will prescribe certain medicines which will control your symptoms. You must keep these medicines handy and use them as per your doctor's advice.

Allergy : Understanding Now and Then

Allergy as a disease condition was recognised by ancient Greek physicians. Allergy is a Greek word which comes from words *Aller* + *erges*, meaning 'altered energy'. A more meaningful insight into the disease process occurred only when Paul Ehrlich identified what is now known as 'Mast Cells' in our body. These 'Mast Cells' play a major role in manifesting symptoms of allergy. Paul Enrlich was eventually awarded the Nobel Prize for his contribution to medical research. The condition of anaphylaxis which is also an allergic response was first explained by *Richet* and *Porter* in the early 20th century. The importance of mast cells in allergic reaction was first explained by *Weiser* in 1957 and later by *J.F. Riley* in 1959.

Even though our understanding of allergy is far more now, the work is still far from being over. Newer insights into this process help doctors reduce the agony of allergic patients. The day is not far, we hope, when 'allergy' will be a trifle ailment.

11

OTHER ALLERGIC DISORDERS AND RHINITIS

Other Allergic Disorders

In the previous chapters, we have learnt a lot about allergic asthma. We have not discussed much of Intrinsic or non-allergic asthma as this book is on 'Allergy' and not on non-allergic pathologies. There are numerous other allergic disorders: (1) seasonal sneezing or hay fever, (2) perennial sneezing or allergic rhinitis, (3) urticaria, (4) allergic ecyema, (5) contact dermatitis, (6) food allergy, (7) drug allergy.

Hay fever and allergic rhinitis mainly affect the nose. Urticaria can be localised or generalised in the body. Eczema affects the skin. Contact dermatitis also is a disorder of the skin. Allergy to drugs and food allergy bring about a generalised allergic reaction. Drug allergy can produce serious reactions which can be life-threatening like Anaphylaxis. It also includes allergy to various vaccines.

We have also included migraine (sick headache) in our section as this disorder has generated a lot of curiosity among patients.

Hay Fever (Seasonal Allergic Rhinitis)

Bouts of sneezing occurring in a particular season is called Seasonal Allergic Rhinitis. Its common name is hay fever. Hay fever does not have any connection with hay. It is the seasonal occurrence of sneezing and running nose with congestion in the nose and itching in the eyes and nose.

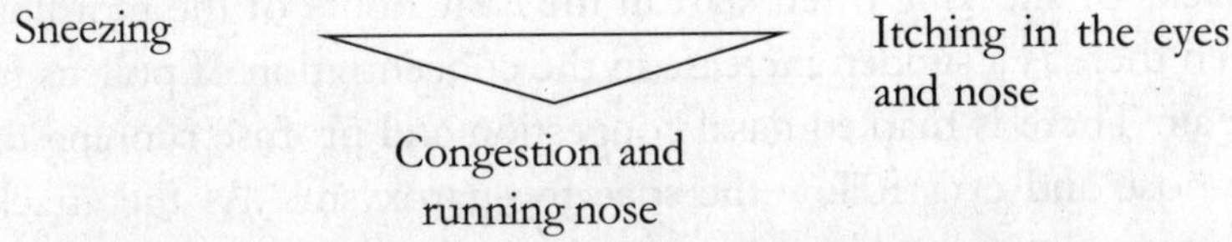

Fig. 11.1 : The Triad of Seasonal Allergic Rhinitis (*Hay Fever*)

The patient has to undergo these symptoms again and again every year in the same season. In the other months, he is normal. It affects both the sexes equally, and occurs in all age groups, but mostly in young people. The symptoms can be mild, moderate or severe. It occurs in those who have inherited an allergic trait from their family. It is caused by an allergic reaction to the pollen emitted by grass and flowers and is often at its worst in UK during the summer. As the pollens to which they are allergic appear in the air in a particular season of the year, the symptoms of the disease occur seasonally.

Symptoms

The onset of sneezing may be gradual or quite sudden depending on the degree of exposure to the particular pollens to which the patient is allergic. When the onset is gradual, the attack is preceded by a mild sensation of itching and burning of the eyes. It may also start a mild irritation in the nose and sometimes there is a itching of the palate inside the mouth.

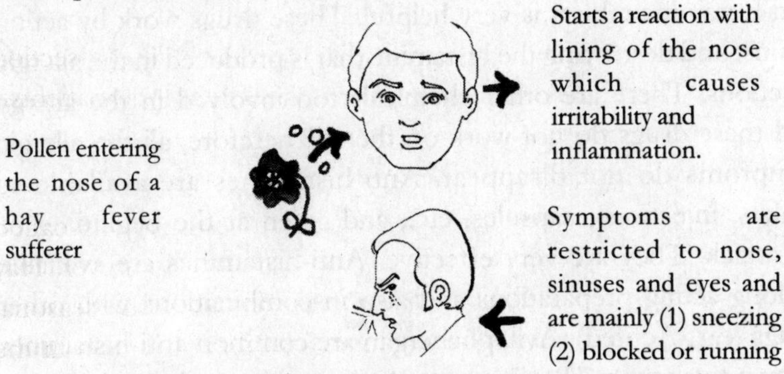

Fig. 11.2 : Hay Fever Manifestation

Attacks of sneezing often start in the early hours of the morning when there is a sudden increase in the concentration of pollens in the air. There is marked nasal congestion and profuse running of the nose and eyes follow the sneezing paroxysms. As the attack progresses, the nasal mucous membrane becomes very sensitive and responds with sneezing to even small stimuli which were previously insignificant. Like strong odours and small amounts of dust, many patients of hay fever also complain of loss of appetite, drowsiness, inertia. This can be attributed even to self-medication with anti-histamines which have a mild sedative effect.

In some patients, there can be seen symptoms of bronchial asthma. They can begin with the onset of the disease or may get included later on. They may accompany only as a cough or may present as a 'cough + bronchospasm' combination. They may continue even after the sneezing has subsided. Diagnosis is done from a detailed history of the patient. To treat the person, one has to first find the nature of pollen or pollens bringing out the disease. Skin tests with pollen extracts, referring to the pollen calendar, matching the pollen with corresponding season gives out the culprit pollen. Once this is done, treating becomes easier.

Treatment is hyposensitisation of the culprit pollens which gives good results in this condition. Symptomatic treatment with anti-histamine tablets is very helpful. These drugs work by acting against and destroying the histamine that is produced in the allergic reactions. There are other chemicals too involved in the allergy and these drugs do not work on them. Therefore, all the allergic symptoms do not disappear. Anti-histamines are available as tablets, injections, capsules, etc., and given at the beginning of an attack. They are very effective. Anti-histamines are available as long acting preparations and also in combinations with other drugs (e.g., Actifed). Avil, phenergan are common anti-histamines known to anyone. They lessen itching, sneezing and running nose, and have been a very good and effective source for symptomatic treatment of hay fever. But they cannot be the cure for hay fever. One has to detect the allergen and subsequently hyposensitise the patient to achieve effective results.

Anti-histamines also have side effects like drowsiness, but nowadays, non-sedative antihistamines are available. One can also take hot tea or coffee with anti-histamines to decrease the drowsiness. Rarely anti-histamines may stimulate the central nervous system and cause irritability, insomnia, etc. They should be given only when needed and not as a routine.

Sneezing attacks in hay fever can be prevented by avoiding the allergen (here it is pollen). (1) One should avoid allergen-exposing activities like gardening, farming, etc. (2) The patient should avoid unwanted outdoor activities during the particular season. (3) Bedroom windows can be kept closed and an air-conditioner can be used.

If left untreated, hay fever can cause permanent damage to the nasal mucosa, and sinuses in the form of chronic infection. The symptoms of hay fever, very severe in a young person, gradually goes down in intensity as the person grows old.

Pollinoses

The term 'Pollinoses' (pollen allergy) is given to a complicated complex of pathological changes in respiratory passages, conjunctival membranes, alimentary tract, nervous system, skin and other organs due to acute allergic inflammations of their tissues in sensitisation to pollen.

Perennial Sneezing (Allergic Rhinitis)

An old magazine has an interesting poem titled "Allergic Rhinitis" which is as follows:

> Catch allergic Rhinitis, the king among colds
> your eyes get as swollen as bulbous petioles

your nose seems to run as fast as the Concorde
and your sneezes could create a Guinness record.

Very soon indeed, you begin to wonder
why someone made that big blunder
of naming the dog, man's friend in chief
when actually it is the unassuming handkerchief

Come stage II and totally blocked is your nose
you can sniff away till you turn the colour of a rose
quite soon you realise there is no other solution
except going around with your mouth wide open

Slowly the phlegm starts to collect in your throat
now it is time to take Amoxycillin as an antidote
you cannot make a sound, the throat is actually dry
but you get better with medicines, by and by.

Now finally its your turn to answer me
do not you dear reader quite agree
that Allergic Rhinitis is a terrible disease
much worse than a fever, headache or wheeze?!

The poem above describes the 'Allergic Rhinitis' in a nutshell and patients of allergic rhinitis cannot have a second opinion about the 'plight' described above.

Allergic rhinitis is not restricted to any particular season and is called Perennial Allergic Rhinitis. The main complaint of most of the patients is blocked or stuffy nose and of a post-nasal discharge. They develop a snore in the night and breathe through the mouth. They develop ear discomfort also as the ear tubes (eustachian tube) opening in the throat get blocked. The mucous membrane of the paranasal sinuses may also get involved in the allergic process and infections causing blockage of the sinus openings and accumulation of secretions. The other manifestations are fever, discharge from ear due to middle ear infection, cough, wheezing, etc. Certain factors such as cold wind, sunlight, dusts, fumes precipitate the onset of symptoms or aggravate the already present symptoms. The symptoms occur more often in the early morning but can continue throughout the day and even the night. Examination of the nose in the acute stage of the disease reveals a swollen, greyish mucous membrane covered with mucous secretion. The swollen mucous membrane obstructs the nasal passages in the chronic stage of the disease. The nasal membrane may be swollen, pearly grey in colour. Mucous and pus are also seen if there is an associated infection. Nasal polyps in the form of a "grape bunch" may also be seen hanging from the mucous membrane and causing a blockage in the nose.

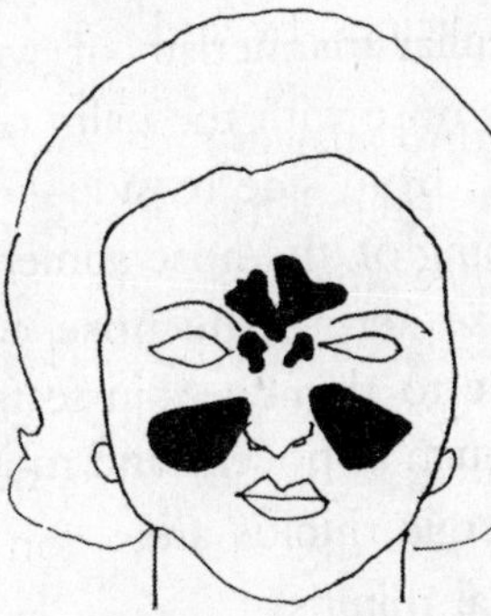

- The sinus cavities are in the skull, between and above the eyes and in cheeks.
- Sinus openings are blocked.

Fig. 11.3 : Location of the Sinuses

The mucous membrane becomes swollen with mucous secretions getting accumulated in the rhinitis.

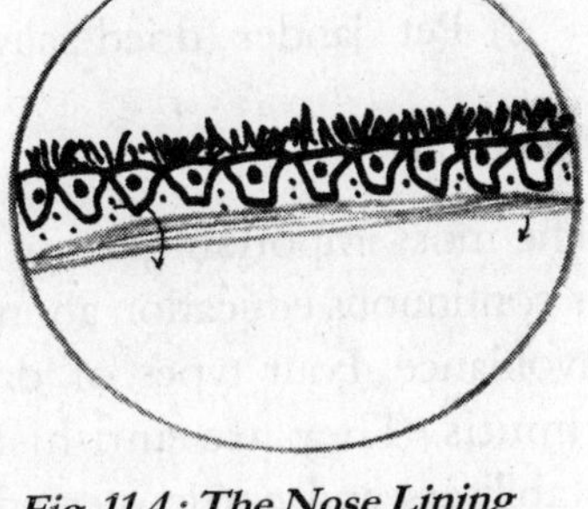

Fig. 11.4 : The Nose Lining

1) In the period of pollinosis, certain children also have food and drug allergy which bothers them only in the pollinating period of the precipitating plants. This phenomenon is called 'Allergic Singergique'.

2) Children with pollinosis (allergic rhinitis) can often be seen rubbing their nose frequently. This characteristic manner is called Allergic Salute. Conjuctiva shows oedema (mild) due to hyperaemia (increased capillary permeability). These two symptoms often are seen together.

Diagnosis and Treatment

The history of the disease is very important. Family history of allergy confirms the diagnosis. Examination of the nose is also very important. Lab examination of nasal secretions may show an increase in eosonophill count (-aWBC). This is an indication of allergy. In children the typical peculiar mannerism of wiping their nose—they elevate the tip of the nose with the palm of the hand and wriggle the nose and mouth from side to side—often confirms the diagnosis. Constant rubbing of the nose sometimes leads to the development of a crease across the nose called 'Allergic Crease'. This also gives a clue to rhinitis. Skin tests are next done with the different allergens such as pollens and moulds.

Common allergens in perennial allergic rhinitis are:

a) Pollen (a culprit more in seasonal rhinitis)
b) Housedust, moulds
c) Pet dander (dried saliva left after grooming)

Medication

The most important part of patient treatment for allergic rhinitis is continuous education about medication, side effects and allergen avoidance. Four types of drugs are widely used to treat allergic rhinitis. They are anti-histamines, decongestants, mast cell stabilisers and corticosteroids. Anti-histamines are antagonists of the body's own histamine that are directed at target in the respiratory mucosa. Since traditional antihistamines were rapidly absorbed with the central nervous system, they caused drowsiness in 10-20 per cent of users. Newer anti-histamines no longer sedate patients and have very few or no side effects. They include Astemizole, Cetrizine, Loratadine. Out of these, Cetrizine, is the only one not metabolised in the liver and is eliminated from the body intact. Astemizole has a slow onset but long duration action. It has a half life of up to 19 days and this makes it ideal for maintenance treatments rather than as needed relief. Recent research has linked some of the new anti-histamines such as Astimizole with cardiac arrhythmia, and they should not be used in conjunction with certain kinds of antibiotics or oral anti-fungal agents nor in the presence of liver disease. Anti-histamines help in perennial rhinitis comparatively less as compared to its role in seasonal rhinitis. Decongestants act by contracting blood vessels in the nose which block airways when they become engorged by allergic reaction. They function well in all kinds of nasal congestion, allergic or non-allergic, but have no effect on the underlying process of rhinitis.

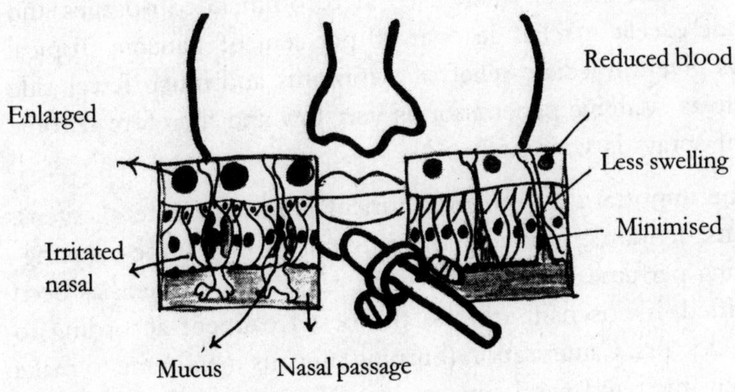

Fig. 11.5 : Action of Decongestant Drugs

Decongestants do not replace more fundamental treatments but rather supplement them. There are topical decongestants that come as sprays or nasal drops—oxymetayoline, xylometayoline, naphayoline—and there are oral decongestants like ephedrine and phenyepropanolamine. Topicals are preferred as they are less prone to systematic side effects such as restlessness, agitation, sleep disturbance, tachycardia, headaches. They are frequently used alongwith anti-histamines and often improve results significantly.

Mast cell stabilisers such as sodium chromoglycate are anti-inflammatory drugs which are effective in mild to moderate cases of rhinitis but less so in the most severe cases. These drugs must be used frequently (4 to 6 times daily) to reduce symptoms and work better against sneezing than stuffed up noses.

Corticosteroids are the most potent of the rhinitis drugs available today. They can be taken orally, through injections or locally. They reduce rhinitis symptoms through a variety of complex mechanisms that are not clearly understood. They inhibit the inflammatory response right where it begins (reduces mast cells close to the surface of epithelia tissue) at the cellular level. They reduce every allergic symptom. Intranasal steroids rarely cause systemic side effects when used at recommended dosages and provide excellent relief in over 90 per cent of patients. Topical sprays give immediate relief of symptoms and much fewer side effects as systemic penetration is very low and therefore chronic use of sprays is very safe.

The important aspect in treatment is to avoid the allergens, pollens, irritants, inducing the rhinitis. Strong fumes, strong-smelling perfumes are to be avoided. Once the allergen has been identified, hyposensitisation is the best treatment according to many doctors. Cauterisation (burning mucous membrane to make it insensitive) and nasal surgery are all best avoided.

Hyposensitisation and drug treatment often help in clearing nasal polyps also. No surgery is needed until the polyps obstruct the nose and interfere with respiration.

A combination of antihistamine plus a decongestant is very effective.

Intranasal steroids are very useful in allergic rhinitis. Topical sprays as mentioned earlier are very safe.

Advantage of nasal sprays can be illustrated as :

Delivers drug directly

↓

Nasal membrane

↓

Very fine particle size

↓

Quickly absorbed

↓

Onset of action almost immediate

↓

Low systemic penetration

↓

Fewer side effects

Currently available topical corticosteroids include Flunsolide, Beclomethasone, Dipropionate and Budesonide. Beginning a course of steroids before the pollen season can prevent cell changes in the nose associated with rhinitis. After two weeks of use, the doses can be reduced to one a day. The aim is to use the minimum effective dose for each patient. Though side effects such as nasal irritation in the first few days may occur in a minority of patients, topical steroids are safer.

Systematic steroids are to be used only in severe cases of rhinitis, with caution. Sometimes given to hay fever, sufferers are particularly efficient at reducing nasal blockage, but have certain unwanted side effects which can be severe and hence systematic steroids are best avoided.

Immunotherapy or Hyposensitisation or Desensitisation

Some doctors consider this very effective. As mentioned earlier, some have claimed 100 per cent cure out of this procedure. It is an expensive, time consuming and risky procedure which seeks to boost the presence of immunoglbulins like G_1 and G_4 which appear to reduce the allergic reactions though it does not make the symptoms disappear completely. Since the procedure requires that the patient be exposed to allergen extracts orally, nasally, directly under the tongue or parentrally (by injection) grave systemic reactions are possible and hence immunotherapy should never be attempted without resuscitation facilities. It has proved useful in treating grass, ragweed, dog and cat allergies, but is useless against dust-mite allergy and not particularly good for hay fever. This treatment modality is altogether too drastic for most rhinitis sufferers, and is rarely used except to treat rhinitis patients with asthmatic symptoms. Again, this view is not agreed by some doctors who prefer this to other modes of treatment.

Surgery in Allergic Rhinitis

Occasionally abnormalities in the nose or sinuses aggravate systems of allergic rhinitis, and in these cases medication may be combined with surgery. Sinus surgery is sometimes used to correct secondary symptoms caused by sinus obstruction. The operation is usually followed by a course of typical corticosteroids.

Recent studies have shown that if patients are provided with appropriate medication, education and instruction, symptoms of allergic rhinitis can be well controlled with minimum impairment of quality of the life.

Next, we must know how to differentiate a common cold from the perennial allergic rhinitis. The following table shows the differences between the two pathologies.

Table 11.1 : Differences between Common Cold and Perennial Allergic Rhinitis

Common Cold	*Perennial Allergic Rhinitis*
Caused by virus and it may have fungal and added bacterial infection.	Allergy-induced pollens, dust, spores, etc. are common allergens.
Begins with malaise, aches and nose and sneezing throughout the year.	Perennial in nature so there is running pain, malaise, appetite, slight fever.
Running nose, sneezing either occur along with the above symptoms or follow them.	Blocked nose and sinuses, middle ear may be infected.
Nasal discharge is at first watery, but later becomes thick. With nasal block, there may be headache, loss of taste sense (Ageusia).	Histological examination of nose reveals swollen mucous membrane, increased mucus secretions. There may be pus in chronic stages if there is an added infection.
Symptoms last for several days to weeks.	
No eosonophills in nasal smear. Skin tests for allergy negative.	Eosonophills are increased. Skin tests for allergy positive.

History

Both of disease and family, examination of nose and nasal examination differentiates the two conditions.

Summary

1. Rhinitis is of two types :

   a) Seasonal (hay fever)—mainly due to pollens.

   b) Perennial—various allergens cause it.

2. Bouts of sneezing, running nose, eye irritation, blocked nose, sinuses constitute the main symptoms.
3. Diagnosis includes history, nasal examination, skin tests for allergy.
4. Hyposensitisation is the main treatment.
5. Anti-histamines,

   Decongestants,

   Corticosteroids, etc.

These form the main agents in symptomatic treatment. Different physicians have different views on the use or non-use of these drugs.

12

ALLERGIC DISORDERS OF SKIN

Urticaria

One of the very common manifestations of allergy is Urticaria. This is more commonly known as Hives. This is experienced by most of the persons at some time of their life. It can be a transient phenomenon (in majority of cases) occurring once or twice. In some, it is seasonal and in few it persists as a chronic phenomenon causing debilitation and misery.

Urticaria can be a localised or generalised phenomenon. It may occur as few spots or it may be confluent. Raised reddish areas of different shapes and sizes appear which cause itching, and this may last for minutes or few hours and disappear without a trace. Fresh urticaria patches can appear later. Urticaria sometimes happens along with swelling of tongue, lips, hands and feet. This condition is called Angio Oedema. This is also called Giant Urticaria. The swelling, redness, etc., in urticaria is due to release of histamine in the tissues.

Causes of Urticaria

1) Physical agents such as cold, heat, sunlight, mechanical pressure.
2) Emotional causes like laughter, anxiety, panic.
3) Food articles such as nuts, seeds, fish, eggs, chicken, citrus fruits, mushrooms.
4) Drugs like aspirin, some antibiotics, laxatives, etc.
5) Systemic diseases like gastroenteritis, appendicitis, tonsillitis.

6) Serious conditions like systemic lupus erythematosus, carcinoma.

7) Insect bites and stings can also cause urticaria.

8) Idiopathic or 'cause unknown' urticaria is also a very common phenomenon.

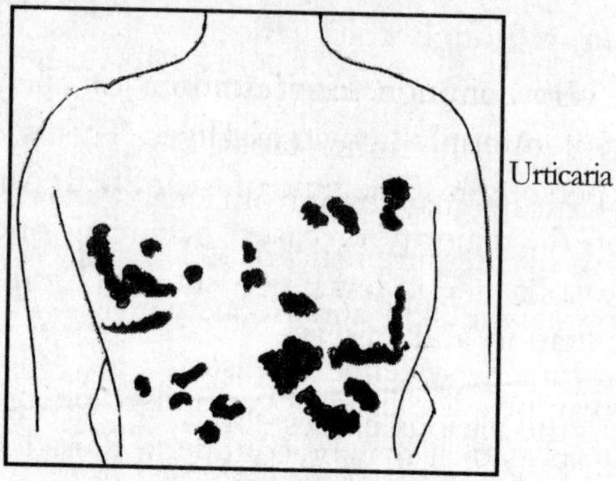

Fig. 12.1 : Onset of Urticaria

Allergic urticaria is caused by substances which enter the body by ingestion, inhalation or injection. The commonest foods in this group include fish, especially shellfish, pork, eggs, strawberries, mushrooms. Drugs are even more common cause of urticaria today, particularly aspirin, penicillin, etc. In this context, the drug probably acts as a histamine liberator. Inhalants are a much less common cause though any of the substances which are capable of causing hay fever, i.e., pollens, dust, horse dander, etc., may on occasion cause urticaria. Vaccines, serums and anti-toxins (particularly tetanus anti-toxin) are examples of substances given by injection. Allergic urticaria also includes the 'gross and widespread oedema' which occurs in a few individuals as a result of stings from mosquitoes, bees and wasps. Intestinal parasites, hydatid cysts are other common allergic causes.

Toxic Urticaria

In this group are cases caused by insect bites, jellyfish stings and stinging nettles (urticaria also has an other name, Nettle Rash). For convenience, the physical urticarias may also be classified here. Urticaria due to light and cold is usually limited to the exposed skin, although cold urticaria may be universal if the temperature is low enough. Light urticaria may be caused by both UV-light and visible light. Heat is a common cause and occasionally urticaria may result from local pressure such as kissing. Another form of pressure urticaria is Dermographism caused by firm stroking of the skin and frequently brought out by drying after a bath. Finally, systemic diseases and certain conditions (as mentioned in the various causes above) can cause urticaria in the form of acute or recurrent whealing.

Nervous Urticaria

Certain cases of urticaria are habitually caused by heat, exercise or emotion, the clinical signs being the onset within a few minutes of a profuse eruption of tiny, equally sized wheals (well defined raised flat lesions, pink at margin and white in centre, caused by liberation of histamine), a few mm in diameter with wide flares. The condition is caused by the liberation of 'acetyl choline', a chemical substance from cholinergic nerves. It is more common in men than women, and occurs in adolescence and early adult life. Urticaria of the normal pattern can also be a psychosomatic disease caused entirely by emotional stimuli, and unassociated with abnormal reactions to heat or exercise.

Urticaria which can present as an acute or chronic manifestation has the following features:

Acute : Wheals appear at irregular intervals for several days, but gradually become less frequent and eventually cease after a week or ten days. This type is usually due to some food or drug.

Chronic : The wheals appear usually about the same time of the day for weeks, months or years. This is the commonest type seen today and it is rare to find a specific cause. Some cases appear to have been caused initially by penicillin.

Signs and Symptoms

Onset is acute, and there may be slight fever. The patient notices intense irritation, then a red blotch appears which rapidly develops into a raised white wheal with red edges. Sometimes the process stops short at the red stage and constitutes the so called Red Urticaria. These lesions persist maximum for a few days. Fresh lesions appear one after the other. The patient scratches, and fresh wheals appear alongwith the scratch marks.

Lewis Triple Response

Reaction of whealing, or Lewis Triple Response, is caused by the liberation of histamine in the skin and follows a multitude of chemical and physical stimuli. Applying a physical/chemical stimuli will produce:

1) Capillary dilation
2) Arteriolar dilatation
3) Fluid escapes from the capillaries due to increased permeability of their walls.

The three responses are:

Red reaction,	The flare,	The wheal.
due to dilation of capillaries	depends on local new mechanisms	raised area on skin is due to increased capillary permeability

In susceptible individuals, even light stimulation, such as drawing a pencil with moderate pressure over the skin of the back, will produce Linear Wheals surrounded by a diffused red halo along the pencils track. In this way, letters or other designs can be embossed upon the skin. This phenomenon is spoken of as 'Dermographism' or 'Factitious Urticaria'.

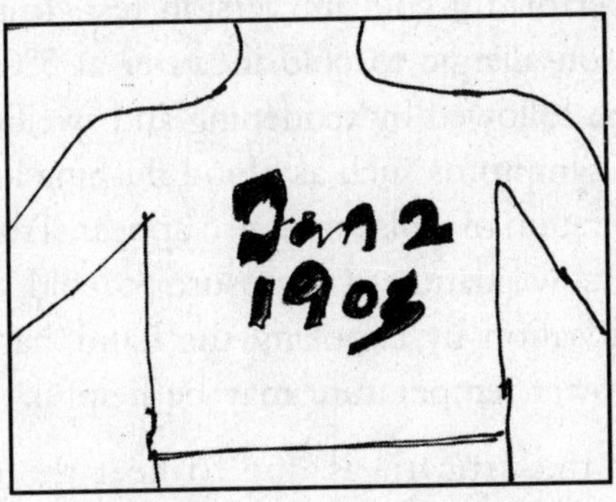

Fig. 12.2 : Linear Wheals

The raised patch is at first clearly demarcated but as time passes, it increases in width and decreases in height, loses its sharpness and finally disappears. This is due to transudation of fluids from the capillaries.

Giant Urticaria

Subcutaneous tissues are involved in this. Attacks usually occur in the early mornings. Circumscribed or diffused swellings one to three inches in diameter are seen. Swellings do not pit on pressure. The skin over them may be of a white or redder (than normal) colour. It may be cold and waxy or red and hot. The usual situations are the face, hands, forearms, genitals, mucous membranes but the swellings can appear anywhere. The swellings may be present in the mouth, tongue, glottis and can cause suffocation. This is important clinically. The swellings reach their full size in a few hours and seldom last for more than 24 hours.

Diagnosis : Urticaria lesions occur in the trunk usually, and individual lesions of urticaria last only for a matter of hours. History is important in diagnosis. Skin tests are of little value.

Prognosis : About 50 per cent of cases clear in less than three months, 10 per cent in a year and 90 per cent in five years.

Before we discuss the treatment we have to determine the underlying cause. If symptoms of urticaria are due to cold, it is necessary to perform a cold immersion test. Immersion of the hand of a person allergic to cold in water at 5°C for five to 10 minutes may be followed by reddening and swelling of the hand. In some cases, symptoms such as blood flushing into the face, fall in BP and accleration of pulse may also appear. Treatment consists primarily of the avoidance of exposure to cold, anti-histamines and hyposensitisation by exposing the hand/hands in water at progressively lower temperature may be helpful.

Similarly if the urticaria is due to heat the case history is important; testing for heat exposure is by using hot water. The patient is asked to put one leg in hot water. Generalised urticaria occurs over the entire body, but the immersed leg merely becomes flushed. Acute reaction to heat is treated using a cooling agent. An attempt to increase tolerance to heat by exposing to higher temperature can be tried gradually.

If the urticaria is due to sunlight, case history and reproduction of lesions by exposing to sunlight (injury or a scar) may develop. Treatment includes change of environment, wearing tinted glasses, staying indoors, avoiding photosensitising substances, coating skin with agents and filtering injurious rays.

If an examination of the stool shows presence of a parasite, proper treatment is needed. Foci of infection in the teeth, tonsils and other places should be treated. Commonly known allergic articles of diet such as eggs, milk, chocolate, chicken, etc., to be avoided and results noted. If there is improvement in symptoms re-administration of eliminated food is carried out one by one and the effect is noted. A one week interval is followed before a new food is added to the diet. Patients are to be warned against taking aspirin, penicillin, laxatives, etc. Suppressive treatment is best carried out with anti-histamines. Ephedrin, adrenaline as a subcutaneous once or twice daily dose, is also followed in some cases. Gentle sedation with pheno or amylobarbitone produces dramatic results in some cases. In certain cases, both acute and chronic, steroid hormones have to be used. Some general instructions for the urticaria patient are:

1) Avoid excessive physical/mental stress.
2) Avoid the physical irritation of the skin.
3) Avoiding the culprit food and medicines if they are the cause of urticaria.

Popular Urticaria It is an allergic urticaria in children as a reaction to

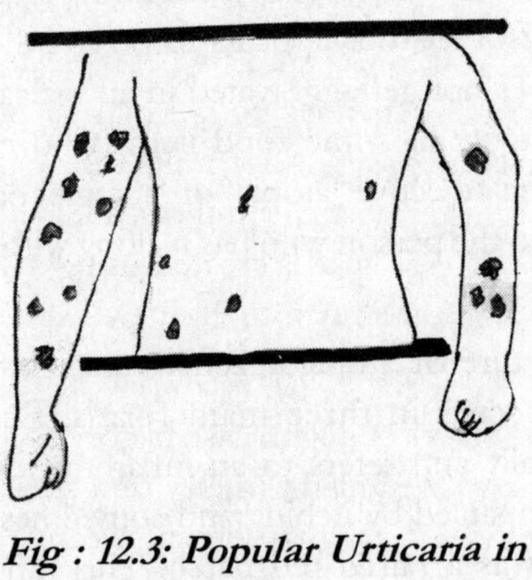

Fig : 12.3: Popular Urticaria in a Child

insect bites (usually animal fleas). The lesions are red blotches or white weals with a central papule (raised, superficial abnormalities of skin). Parasites are to be destroyed with disinfectants and the child is treated with anti-histamines, etc. One characteristic feature of this popular urticaria is that often they are found on extensor aspect of the limbs.

Allergic Eczema

What is eczema ? When some external agent inflames the skin a series of highly characteristic changes develop in the epidermis (the top layer of skin) to which the term eczema is applied. Allergic eczema appears in individuals who have a genetic trait for allergy. The person may have one or two manifestations of allergy in him apart from eczema like, for example, he may have asthma or hay fever. In other words, the type of eczema which frequently occurs in combination with conditions like urticaria, hay fever, asthma is called Atopic or Allergic Eczema. The more severe the eczema the more likely is the individual to suffer from the related allergic conditions and in the severest cases, the incidence of asthma is approximately 50 per cent, urticaria 10 per cent and hay fever 5 per cent. There is a marked familial incidence of all these conditions and the worst cases occur when both parents are atopic. The basis of the disorder thus appears to be an inherited genetic defect. Eczema does not get aggravated in an urticaria patient (if he has hypersensitivity to some food item) who consumes the allergic food. So the adjective 'atopic' or 'allergic' does not apply to the eczema but to the person who has it along with other allergic conditions.

The clinical picture of atopic eczema varies with the age of the patient and occurs in three main forms. Eczema means 'bubbling up' literally and refers to an inflammation of the skin that is often accompanied by itching and sometimes blisters. The eczema rash starts as a raised red patch. This rapidly develops into blisters and these blisters weep. Ultimately they crust over. The open sores are very itchy and may well become infected. If left untreated, the skin becomes thicker and may begin to resemble cracked leather.

The three main forms of atopic eczema :

1) *Infantile Atopic Eczema (Infantile Eczema)*

This begins about the third month of life, on the cheeks, soon spreading to the forehead and chin but sparing the skin around the mouth, nose and eyes. It may remain limited to these parts or it may extend to the scalp, limbs, trunk. The affected skin is red and rough with minute cracks oozing serum or closely set vessicles appear on a hot, red, swollen surface. Itching is great, and rubbing and scratching quickly lead to loss of the horny layer and exposure of a weeping surface. As the serum dries, this becomes crusted. The disease varies from time to time having a great tendency to relapse when nearly well. The child is usually very fretful at night. In the majority of cases, the condition clears up towards the end of the third year.

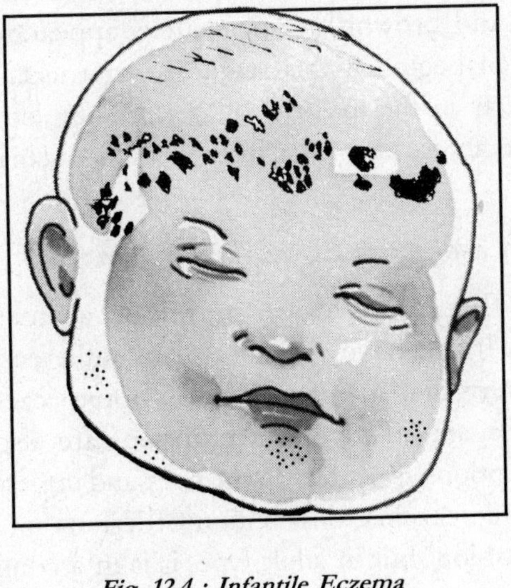

Fig. 12.4 : Infantile Eczema

2) *Atopic Eczema of Childhood (Flexural Eczema)*

This may follow straight on from infantile eczema or it can appear without the preceding infantile phase. The antecubital (in the hand) and the popliteal (in the leg) fossae are the sites where the lesions are seen. They can be also seen on the wrist, groin and on the ankles. To begin with the lesions are papular, scaly with little excoriations.

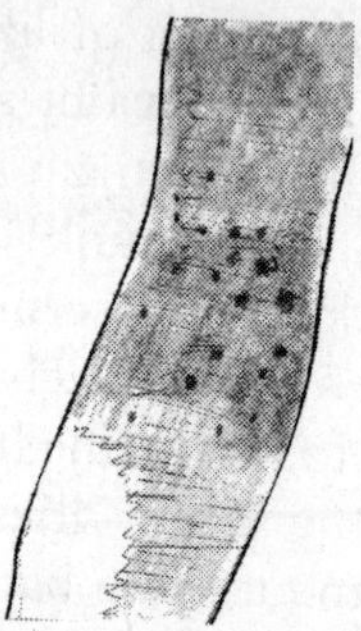

Fig. 12.5 : Atopic Eczema of Children

Later these become pigmented. There are periods of quiescence followed by periods of intense irritation. Lichenification (thickening and brownish/violet patchy appearance) continues. Asthma often begins at this stage. Eczema usually clears at or before puberty in the majority of cases. The pictures shows the thickening in antecubital fossa of the hand in a childhood eczema case.

3) *Adolescence and Atopic Eczema Besniers Prurigo.*

This follows flexural eczema with or without an intervening period of freedom. It can have a history of infantile eczema or rarely present as very first manifestation of atopic eczema. The limb flexures are again affected, but eruptions are also seen on the face with eruptions spreading to the neck and upper half of trunk. In the infantile eczema, distribution of lesions on face was in a 'mask-like fashion' but in adult type, it is in a confluent fashion.

It will be localised in mild cases, but will be universal in distribution in severe cases. There is papules, lichenification (thickening) and pigmentation. In severe cases, there is lot of itching, the skin is pale, dry and rough. The more severely affected of the patients do not perspire freely owing to the occlusion of the sweat ducts. Finally, 10 per cent of affected cases develop Juveni Cataract.

Atopic eczema in all its stages is particularly prone to the aggravating and perpetuating factors common to all eczematous conditions: (1) Scratching, rubbing, etc., to relieve itching, washing, etc., aggravate it. (2) Warmth, perspiration, etc., increase it. (3) Psychological factors also aggravate it. (4) Woollen clothing, cold, drying and chapping weather, emotional stress (as mentioned already) all aggravate the condition. For instance, most patients are worse in the winter and better in the summer assuming they do not become overheated, and exacerbations associated with school, examinations, marriage and childbirth are commonplace. These features must be constantly borne in mind with regard to treatment.

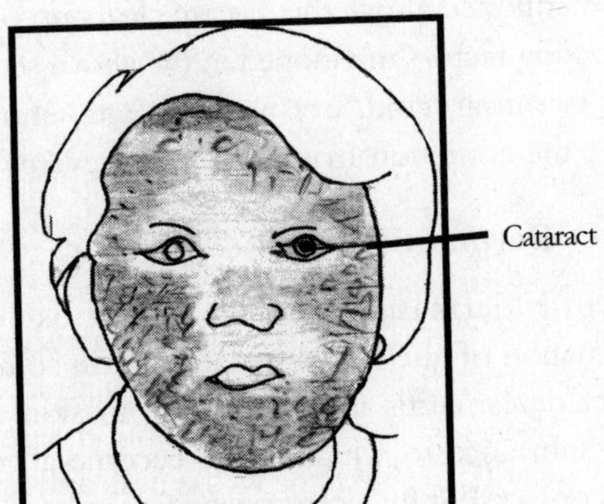

Fig. 12.6 : Atopic Eczema

Diagnosis : In all stages, the distribution of the eruption is the most important diagnostic feature, the family and allergic history and finally the severe itching during and after childhood leading to lichenification. Some conditions have to be distinguished from atopic eczema for proper diagnosis. They are : (1) severe napkin dermatitis in infants with secondary spread can be distinguished by the site of onset and absence of itching. (2) In adults Seborrhoeic Eczema affects mainly the body flexures as opposed to those of the limbs, and lichenification is uncommon. (3) Eczematous determatitis is much more localised although a mild case of atopic eczema limited to the hands may at first be mistaken for dermatitis.

Prognosis: The general tendency in all the stages is towards recovery. The milder the eczema the fewer the related conditions and the less the family history the better is the prognosis. On the other hand, if cases of infantile eczema are severe enough to be admitted to hospital only about a third clear up by the age three while eczema is still present at puberty in a half and after the age of 20 in a quarter.

As mentioned above the disease clears up on its own generally. Aggravating factors mentioned in the above section like emotional stress, sweating, cold, dry weather, etc., should be avoided to prevent the condition from becoming severe.

Contact Dermatitis

The word 'dermatitis' is used almost exclusively to denote inflammation of the skin originating from some external sources. Contact determatitis is the reaction in skin caused by contact with a substance to which it has become allergic because of an earlier contact. For the occurrence of contact dermatitis, an allergic background of the person concerned is not necessary. Prolonged and recurrent contact is necessary to initiate this reaction. The cause of dermatitis can be a solid, liquid or gas. It can be caused by even small quantities of a substance. Some substances are more likely to cause it than others. The sexes are equally affected. There is no familial or racial predisposition. It is uncommon in childhood and old age. This is because contact with potential allergens or irritants occurs less frequently in these age groups. Contact dermatitis cases are on the increase as more and more people are exposed to newer and larger number of drugs and chemicals. The substances that cause contact dermatitis either produce irritation of the skin because of their inherent chemical nature or are non-irritating in themselves and yet cause allergic reactions. The more concentrated a substance is the more readily it excites an allergic response. The liability of a person to become sensitive to the substances mentioned below varies from person to person. Rubber, hair dyes, oils and soaps; chemicals like sulphonamides; antibiotics like penicillin; plant and plant products—all these can cause dermatitis.

The dermatitis is mediated by two completely separate mechanisms referred to as Allergy and Primary Irritation:

1) *Allergic Dermatitis* : In this the causative substance must come in contact with the outside of the skin. Intradermal injection, inhalation or ingestion will not elicit a reaction. Substances causing allergic dermatitis are called Sensitisers. They may be single elements such as nickel, highly complex chemicals such as resins and plastics or even bacterial proteins. In every case, they are absorbed into the epidermis where they become conjugated with epidermal protein. Not until this conjugation has taken place do they become antigen, i.e., capable of provoking formation of antibody. Then they travel via the lymphatics to lymph glands where the antibody formation takes place. Antibodies enter the circulation in association with W.B.C.'s. Once they enter the skin, the antibodies gets fixed to the epidermal cells, and by combination with fresh antigen provokes an

eczematous (not urticarial) reaction. Where it is thought that a case of dermatitis is allergic in origin, the suspected substance must be placed on the surface of the skin. The resulting reaction may begin in 12 hours, reach peak in 48 hours. Sometimes it takes a week. Hence this is called 'delayed type' of allergy. This is a 'cutaneous allergy' response.

2) *Primary Irritant Dermatitis :* This is not produced by an antigen antibody, reaction but by a direct irritant effect on the epidermal cells. A primary irritant is defined as a substance which will produce dermatitis in anybody if allowed to act for a sufficient time at sufficient concentration. Individual susceptibility however varies enormously. For instance, one common type of primary irritant dermatitis results from the effect of household washing (housewives dermatitis) but whereas one woman will develop the condition shortly after her first baby is born, due to increase in washing, another may have 10 children and never develop it. Once the primary irritant dermatitis has developed, other areas of skin are no more susceptible to the substance than they were before in contradistinction to allergic dermatitis. On the other hand, primary irritant dermatitis is more difficult to cure and more prone to persist than allergic dermatitis.

Symptoms : One of the most important characteristic of this dermatitis is its tendency to persist after the original cause is removed. The involved skin is peculiarly prone to further irritation and minor traumata which would have no effect on normal skin are quite sufficient to perpetuate dermatitis. The time interval between the first contact and for sensilisation of the skin to develop symptoms with the substance varies from one to three weeks. Once the sensitisation has developed, the subsequent contact leads to the appearance of the skin lesion within hours. The first symptom is itching, localised to area of contact though it may spread to adjacent areas as well. The itching can make the patient scratch that hastens the skin reaction which is to follow. A redness is first noted in the affected area which progresses to the stage of small raised lesions with fluid in them. These are the papules and vesicles. In the chronic stage, there is confluence of lesions leading to thickening of skin, bacterial infection and pus formation. As the disease progresses, there is no more localisation; no demarcation between normal and affected areas of skin. Even contact of the oozing secretions with the other areas produce lesions as the whole skin has been sensitised. The severity and course of disease depends on sensitisation potential of the patient's skin and the amount of contact. The parts of the body affected are exposed to areas. The region or part of the skin involved assists in determining the causative factor.

Leathers, rubber., fabrics, dyes, etc.	—	Involve feet, lower extremities; trunk, etc.
Cosmetics	—	Face/armpit
Toys	—	Lesions on hands, upper extremities
Metals	—	When articles made of metals which produce allergy in the individual comes in contact with skin, dermatitis ensues, depending on the area in contact.

Secondary Factors : Scratching, trauma and other such factors. Let us discuss the causative factors in detail. The number of substances capable of causing dermatitis is enormous and in a highly civilised and scientifically oriented society, is being added to daily. For descriptive purposes, however, they may be grouped under five headings:

1) *Plants Allergy*: Primary irritant dermatitis is usually limited to children and may be caused by buttercups, daisies, wall flowers. It affects the exposed areas. Sometimes it is severe enough to

cause Bullae (blisters containing serum), for instance, on the lips of children who chew buttercup stalks. At other times, it consists of closely set, small red papules scattered over fingers, hands, forearms. The majority of cases of plant dermatitis, however, occur in adults who have become sensitised (allergic dermatitis). The commonest causes are chrysanthemums, primulas, narcissi, daffodils, carrots, celery, hops, peels of oranges and lemons, bulbs of tulips, hyacinths, garlic, onions. Plant products can also cause dermatitis. Marking nut, henna, calotropis, mango, etc., can also produce symptoms of dermatitis. The exposed skin is usually involved and the reaction can be sudden and intense. In the case of primulas there can be oedema of eyelids. If it is due to handling of bulbs, it can lead to dry fissuring of pulps of thumbs/fingers.

Parthenium Allergy is also an important phenomenon. Parthenium, a weed native to South and Central America, got accidentally introduced in India in 1956. The weed was first detected in Pune. It is found in abundance in Maharashtra, UP, Jammu and Kashmir, and Karnataka. It can grow in any type of soil.

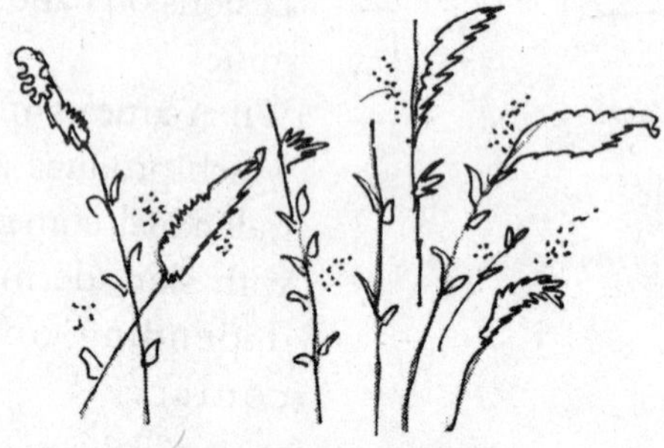

Fig. 12.7 : Parthenium

It is commonly known as 'gajar ghas' (carrot weed). The weed can complete four lifecycles in one year. The initial symptoms are itching around sides of neck and face. Itching then spreads from face to neck, elbows, knees and may involve the whole body. Swelling of skin and watery discharge oozing out of the lesions are the next symptoms. The skin gradually becomes thick and dark. Scratching starts leaving marks. Continued itching can be frustrating. Parthenin, a chemical component, has been found to be the chief culprit for these reactions. This is found in leaves and in fine hair present in the stem.

Diagnosis: Patch test is very important in diagnosis. Application of the suspected substance to the skin for 48 hours is known as a Patch Test. Its only use is in the diagnosis of allergic contact dermatitis since primary irritant substances will normally produce inflammation when left in contact with the skin for this length of time. In the case of a soluble substance, lint is soaked in a suitable solution usually between 1 and 5 per cent strength and test is carried out. A solid, such as clothing, may be placed directly on the skin or, in the case of wood, rubber, plastics, grated and moistened and then applied on lint. Elastoplast is the best adhesive for individuals sensitive to sellotape. Although the majority of positive results are seen in 48 hours, a reaction may only become apparent up to five days after the patch is removed. A positive result in shown by an area of eczema in the skin tested. False positive and false negative results can occur for various complex reasons. Patch test should be looked upon only as a confirmatory test which may add the final piece of evidence to incriminate a substance already suspected on clinical grounds of having caused allergic dermatitis.

The patch test described above can be done in plant allergy. The cause and effect relationship in case of parthenium and allergic reaction is well demonstrated by the patch test. Either crude plants or the antigenic extracts prepared from plant parts are used. Treatment includes: avoiding contact

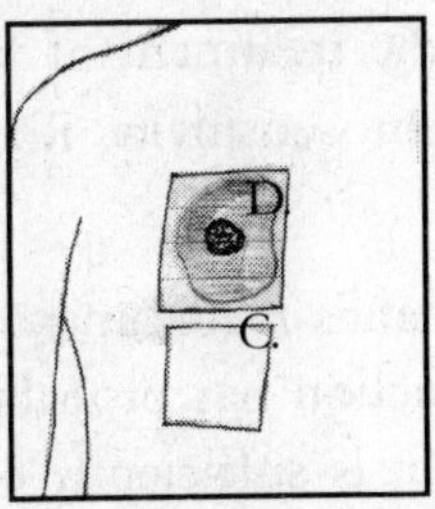

Fig. 12.8 : Positive Patch Test to Hair Dye (The lower square marks the control patch.)

with plant directly or indirectly. Anti-histamines and steroids are not very effective in parthenium allergy. In this allergy, removing the patient from the area infested with parthenium weeds makes him well even without medications. Weedicides and other anti-weed measures are used to destroy such weeds.

2) Vegetable Allery: Having discussed the plant allergies, we can now discuss allergy to vegetable products. The black juice of the marking nut (*Semecarpus anacardium*) produces vesicles on skin. The juice of marking nut known as *Bhilawa* is used by washerman to put identity mark on laundry clothes. When such clothes are worn, it can produce dermatitis by contact. Application of henna can lead to sensitisation in some cases. Small skin eruptions which are oozing are seen on palms/soles. Henna powder can also contact dermatitis of the whole face. The latex which oozes out of calotropis is a strong irritant to skin. When used by some people to treat some skin diseases, it may cause eruptions, bullae or even ulcers. Mango plant and juice of its fruit also produce allergic lesions sometimes on the skin. The juice of unripe fruit, its peel also cause allergy. Mango dermatitis is more common among foreigners than among local population. A vegetable called zamikand (*Amorphophallus companulatus*) also causes itching, redness, urticaria in housewives handling it. It can be prevented from causing allergy by applying a vegetable oil on the hands before handling it. The seeds of *Babchi* (*Psoralea corylifolia*) (which yields an essential oil used in the treatment of leucoderma) also cause contact dermatitis and phtosensitivity. Redness, blisters are seen in sensitive individuals.

3) Drug Allergy: 'Dermatitis medicamentosa' is a common drug allergy. An occasional reaction has probably occurred with every known medicament but it is sufficiently common with some to cause their use as local applications to be abandoned. The most

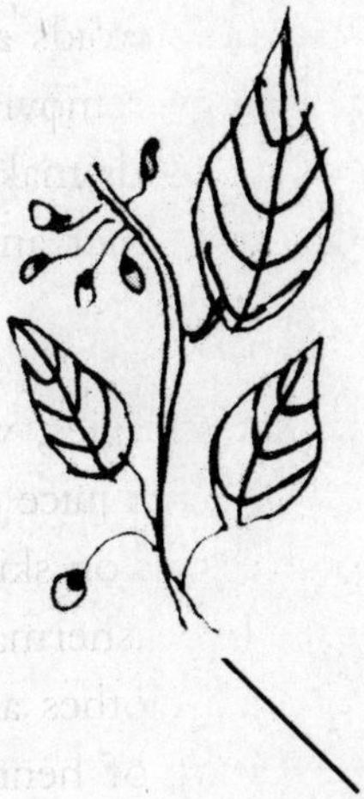

Fig. 12.9 : Marking Nut

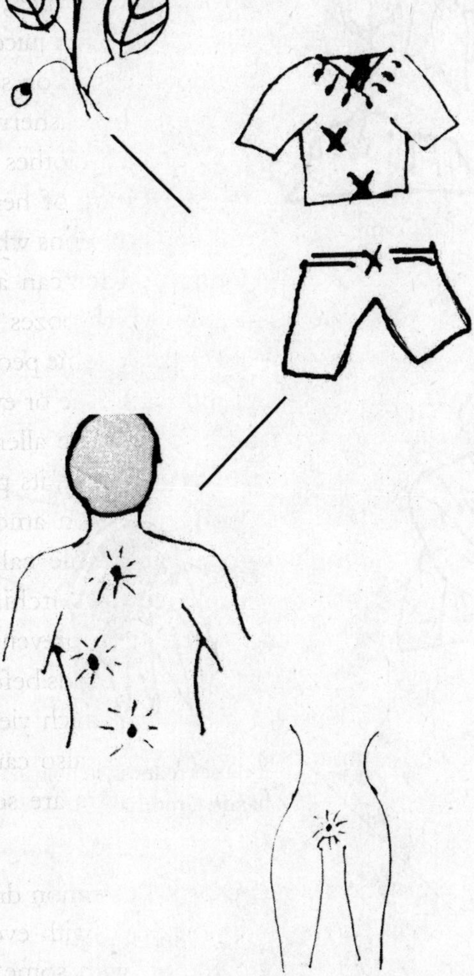

·lryman's mark for identity

Fig. 12.11 : Wearing clothes with dermatitis on strategic locations

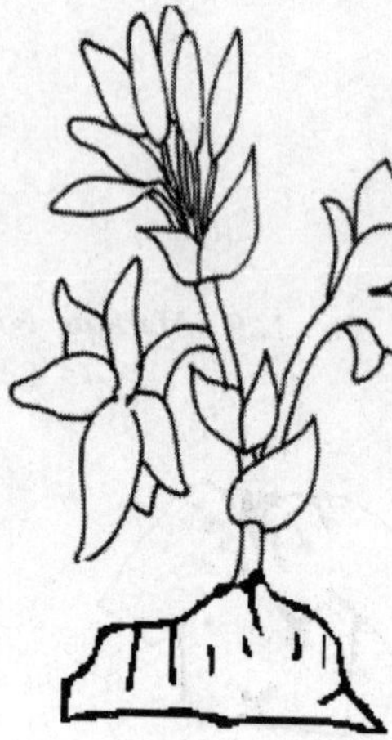

Yam

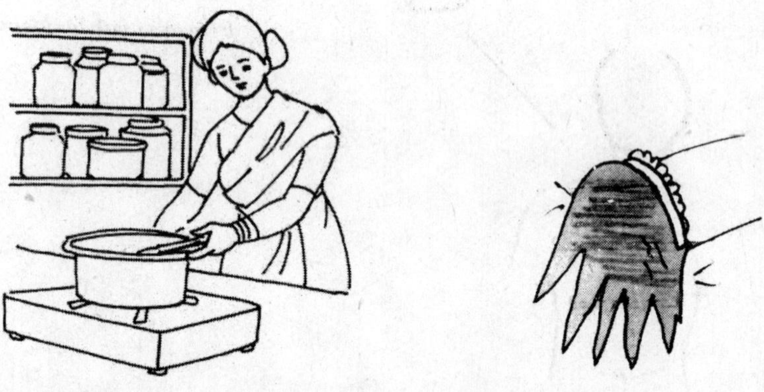

it causes redness, itching in hands; Urticaria

A housewife handling it in kitchen; if she is sensitive

Fig. 12.12 : Yam and Allergies caused by It

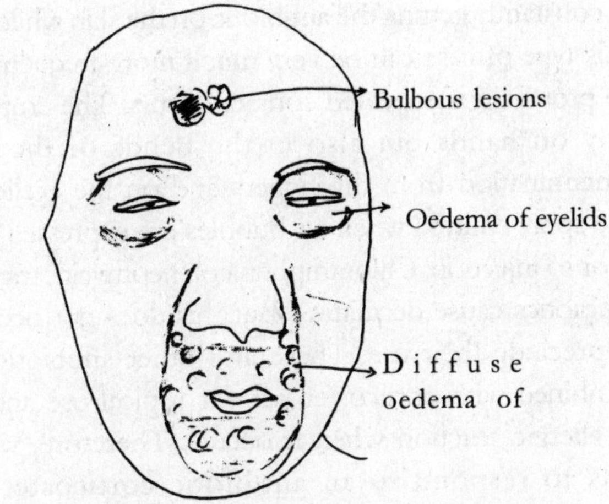

Fig. 12.13 : Plant Dermatitis

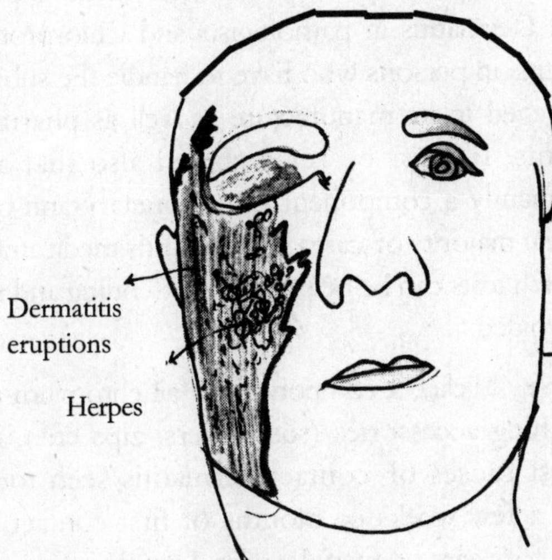

Fig. 12.14 : Dermatitis Medicamentosa

important of these are the sulphonamides, penicillin, streptomycin, procaine group of local anaesthetics and anti-histamines. Cases of penicillin dermatitis have occurred in nurses and doctors as a result of constantly getting the antibiotic on the skin while giving injections. This type of case can be very much more frequent and severe with streptomycin if repeated contact occurs. The eruption appears not only on hands but also in the bends of the elbows, due to contamination from the fingers and on the eyelids caused by the fine spray emitted when air bubbles are expressed from the syringe prior to injection. Chloramphenicol, neomycin, framycetin are other antibiotics cause dermatitis. But this does not occur often enough to preclude their use. These and other antibiotics are frequently combined with corticosteroids for topical use and this may mark an allergic reaction when it occurs. Therefore, when a condition fails to respond to an antibiotic corticosteroid mixture in circumstances in which improvement normally follows, it should always be suspected that sensitisation has occurred and another antibiotic substituted. Largely Procaine Dermatitis is seen in dentists, Formalin Dermatitis in pathologists and Chlorpromazine (Largactil) Dermatitis in persons who have to handle the substance, namely, those engaged in its manufacture as well as pharmacists, nurses and patients. It must be remembered also that a local anaesthetic is frequently a component of proprietary anti-pruritic ointments. The great majority of cases of dermatitis medicamentosa are allergic, and patch tests can be helpful. The offending and related drugs are to be avoided.

4) *Clothing Allergy* : Nickel, a component of all chromium-plated jewellery and clothing accessories (suspenders, zips etc.), is one of the commonest causes of contact dermatitis seen today. It may occur within a few weeks or months of first contact but is frequently delayed for years or even decades. Largely it may appear in all sites of contact simultaneously or consecutively over a period of months. In about three-quarters of the patients other areas not in contact with nickel subsequently become involved, the commonest being the antecubital fossae (hand region) and the eyelids.

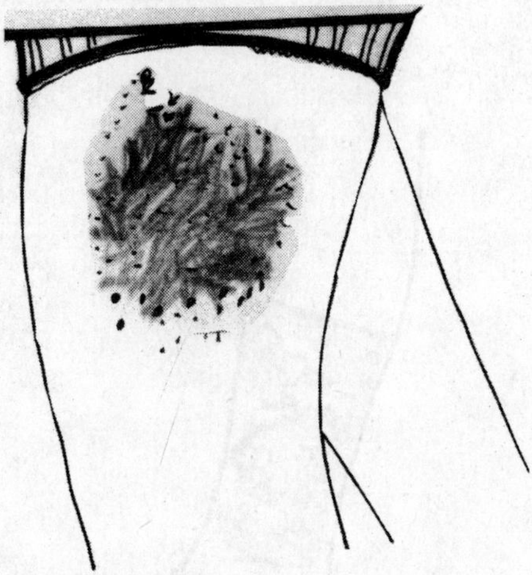

Fig. 12.15 : Suspender Dermatitis

Since patients sometimes seek advice concerning these secondary manifestations without informing the doctor of the primary eruption, a history of nickel sensitivity should always be sought when dealing with obscure eczematous eruptions. Not all cases of Suspender Dermatitis are due to nickel, however, some of the patients being sensitive to rubber. This substance also causes dermatitis when present in the form of corsets and other articles of clothing, contraceptives and gloves.

Dermatitis from clothes is usually due to the dye with which they are coloured. This is particularly so with furs and man- made fabrics (nylon, etc.) since they are dyed with synthetic dyes, more potent sensitisers than vegetable dyes. Fur Dermatitis is seen on the sides of the neck and chin. Nylon Stocking Dermatitis is on the dorsal aspects of toes and feet, the popliteal fossae (calf region) and the upper inner thighs, while in the case of dyed nylon hairnets it occurs at the scalp margin above the ears and at the back of the head. Shoe Dermatitis is usually due to chemical additives in leather or rubber, incorporated to preserve the fabric.

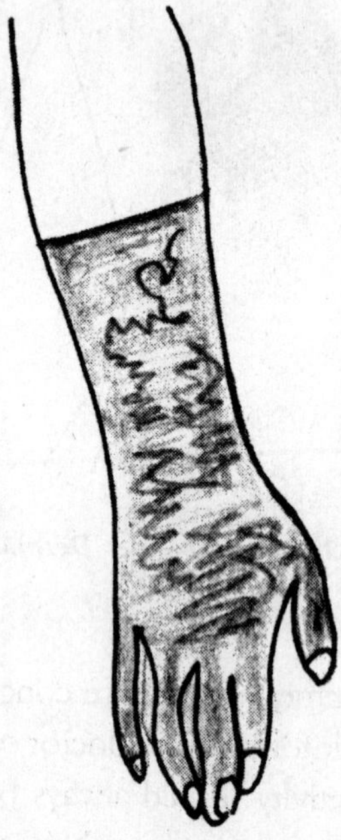

Fig. 12.16 : **Rubber Dermatitis**

5) Cosmetics Allergy: Lipstick Dermatitis is usually limited to the vermilion of the lips, sparing both the adjacent skin and the mucosa and presents as swelling, scaling, cracking or dryness. It accounts for 50 per cent of all cases of Cosmetic Dermatitis and is due to the dye Eosin. Non-allergic lipsticks containing some other colouring agents are now freely available. Nail varnish is the second commonest cause of cosmetic dermatitis. The most notable feature of this is that it does not occur on fingers or hands, but on the more vulnerable skin of the face, neck and particularly eyelids. The site depends on the exact habits of sleep and posture

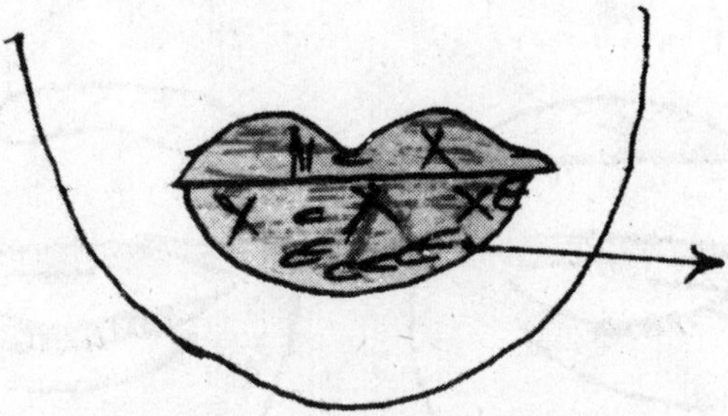

Fig. 12.17 : Lipstic Dermatitis

whereby the nails are brought into contact with the face. Non-allergic nail varnishes are also available. Hairdye Dermatitis usually caused by paraphenylene diamine may be very severe affecting the face more than the scalp with gross swelling of the eyelids and sometimes dissemination over trunks and limbs.

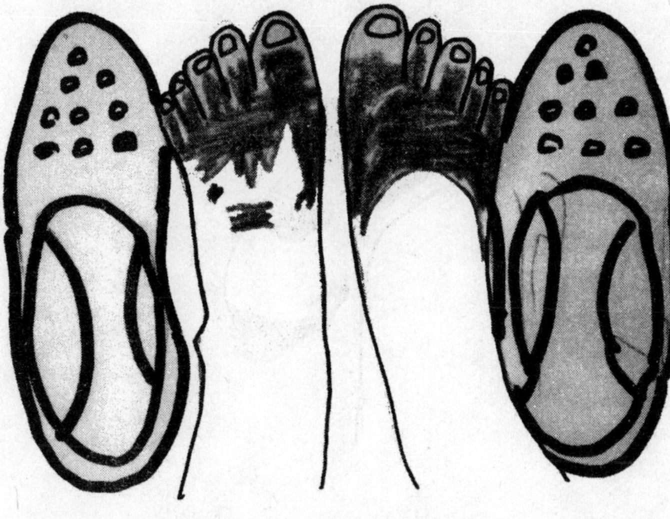

Fig. 12.18 : Shoe Dermatitis

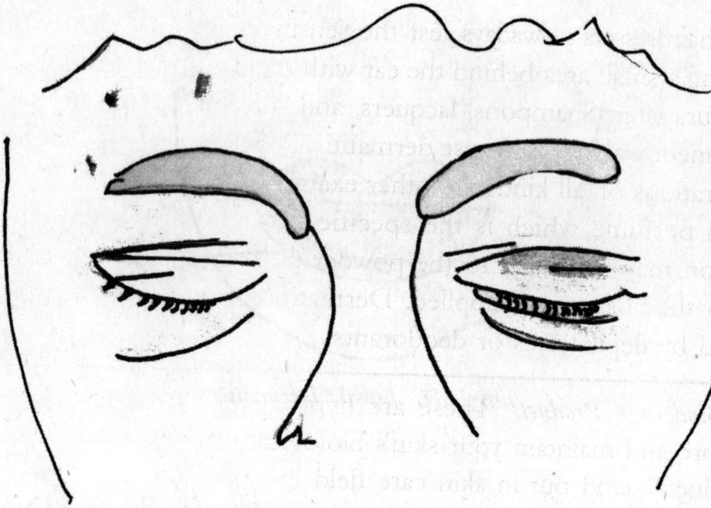

Fig. 12.19 : Dermatitis of Eyelids caused by Nail Varnish

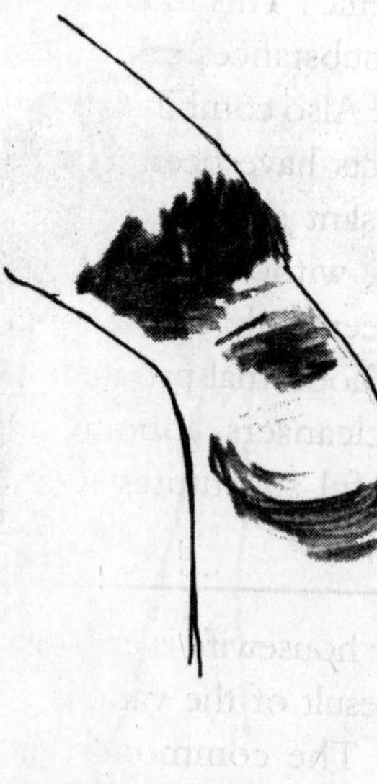

Fig. 12.20 : Axillary dermatitis due to Dye in Clothing

Most hairdressers nowadays test the sensitivity of their clients by painting a small area behind the ear with the dye and examining it 24 hours later. Shampoos, lacquers, and substances used in cold permanent waxing also cause dermatitis. Powders, rouge, cosmetic preparations of all kinds are other examples. Frequently, it is the added perfume which is the specific factor or sometimes the reaction may be traced to the powder puff or rubber pad with which the cosmetic is applied. Dermatitis of the axilla may be caused by depilatories or deodorants.

Biodermal Products: These are hypo-allergic products that restore and maintain your skin's biological balance. Biodermal products stand out in skin care field in an extraordinary way. These products make use of only natural ingredients. Substances that occur naturally in the human body are used in biodermal products. In this way, products are created and they prevent skin irritation and allergic reactions. These products are an answer to skin problems. Descriptions of biodermal products use the term 'hypo-allergenic'. This indicates that all biodermal products contain natural substances known to carry a minimal risk of allergy or irritation. Also combinations of the ingredients used in biodermal products have been tested in test panels to avoid allergic and unpleasant skin reactions. Biodermal hypo-allergenic products have, without exception, been tested on the skin of human volunteers only. These can be used by people with allergic tendencies. Biodermal products include perfumes, hand/body creams, biocleansers, lotions and day and night cream. These can be useful substitutes to the allergy-causing cosmetics in allergic subjects.

Household Dermatitis: The housewife is exposed to a large number of potential irritants as a result of the various stains, polishes and cleaning agents she uses. The commonest cause of dermatitis however is detergents.

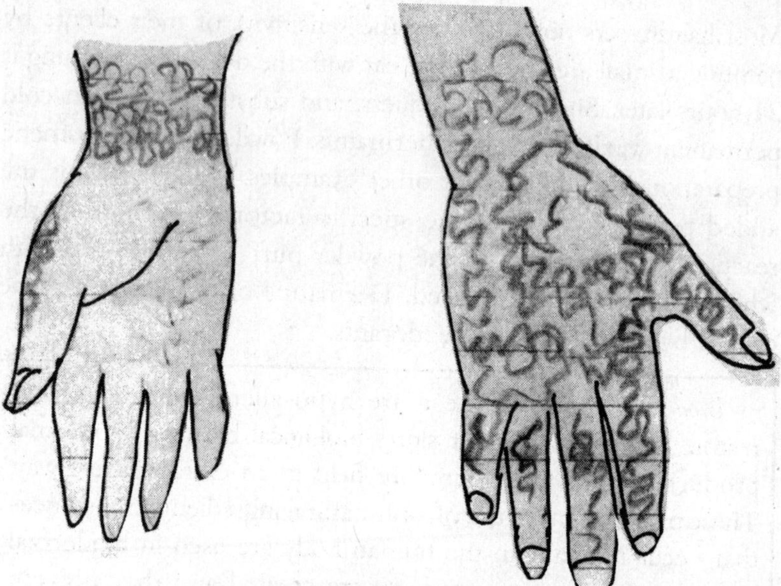

Fig. 12.21 : Household Dermatitis affecting Hands

In modern usage a detergent is a substance used in solution for cleansing and includes soap and synthetic detergents. Both these groups of substances are primary irritants and will cause dermatitis in everyone if used in sufficient strength for long enough. There is no direct evidence that synthetic detergents are more prone to cause dermatitis than soaps, assuming that they are used in reasonable concentrations. Detergents produce dermatitis by direct penetration of the horny layer of skin and by their general *defatting action*, the latter being enhanced by cold winter weather. There is wide individual variation, and dermatitis may occur soon after beginning normal household duty or after a long lifetime of floor scrubbing. In a number of cases, the eruption begins under a ring due to an accumulation of detergent at this site where it remains despite rinsing. Usually it begins as a drying, flaking and fissuring on the sides and backs of the fingers, the backs of the hands and fronts of the wrists or forearms, becoming in a matter of weeks or months vesicular and weeping. Once fully developed, it tends to persist for a considerable time in spite of treatment. Subsequently recurrences are common and there is no doubt that emotional factors play a large part in their occurrence.

Industrial Dermatitis : Less than a fifth of all cases of Industrial Dermatitis are allergic, the commonest causes of which are plants, rubber, dyes, resins, glues and all types of chemicals. Certain hardwoods such as rosewood, Iroko and teak may cause allergic dermatitis especially in the form of sawdust. Resins are used largely in the plastic industry, the newly introduced Epoxy resins being potent sensitisers. Vegetable glues are harmless, but formaldehyde containing synthetic glues used in the furniture and cabinet making trades are sensitisers. Developers used in photography, chrome and nickel contacted in plating and a host of chemicals found in the chemical and munition industries are all capable of causing allergic dermatitis. Sensitisation to the minute amount of chrome present in cement accompanies, and may be one of the causes of Cement Dermatitis. Among the commonest causes of primary irritant Industrial Dermatitis is the simple abrasive effect of dust from such sources as coal, stone, brick and cement. Slightly more sophisticated but in the same context is the action of glass wool. Soaps vigorously used for cleansing may *cause* rather than prevent dermatitis. Detergents are also the irritant factors responsible for dermatitis caused by soluble or cutting oils used to aid cutting and cooling by lathe operators. Diesel oil may cause dermatitis for the same reason. More powerful agents which are sometimes also unwisely used for cleansing the skin beside their more usual industrial uses are paraffin, white spirit, turpentine, thinners and petrol.

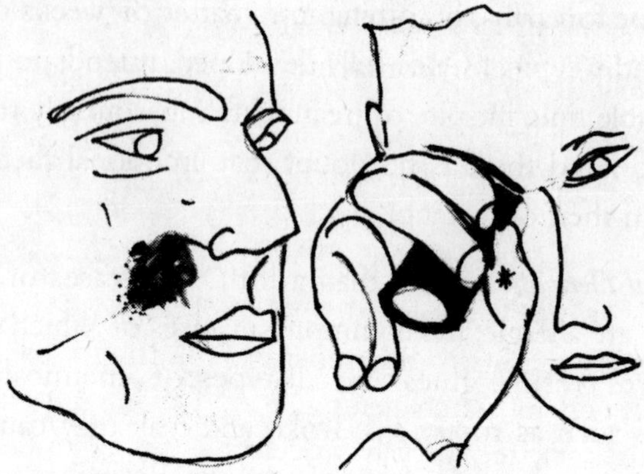

Fig. 12.22 : Industrial Dermatitis

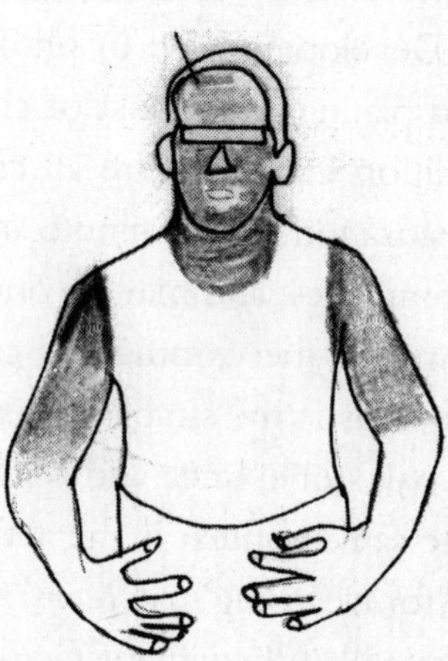

Fig. 12.23 : Photo Dermatitis

The whole skin might have become sensitised but the eruption only occurs in areas exposed to light. Halogenated phenols, such as Tetrachlorsalicylanilide and Bithionol which may be added to soap as an atiseptice agent, act in this way. Even though the patient washes all over with soap, the dermatitis is limited to the exposed areas. Medicaments which can cause Photo Dermatitis are sulphanamides/chlorpromazine (Largaetil); promethazine (Phenergan).

Treatment for Contact Dermatitis: As mentioned in the section on plant and drug dermatitis, the first essential is to remove the patient from contact with the causative substance. In the case of allergic dermatitis, this will probably have to be permanent although occasionally the sensitivity is lost over the years as demonstrated by patch testing. In the case of primary irritant dermatitis once recovery has occurred, some modified form of contact may usually be allowed. For example, women who have suffered from detergent dermatitis may return to household washing so long as prolonged immersion of the hands is avoided and the detergent solution is as weak as is practicable. Even in the primary irritant group, however, avoidance may have to be lifelong.

When suitable substitutes are available, they should be provided, for instance, non-allergic cosmetics and plastics suspenders. In the case of the housewife, however, future contact with detergents cannot be avoided except by protective measures. Cotton or nylon gloves should be worn day and night during the early stages of treatment, and waterproof gloves superimposed for wet work. Later such strict precautions may be relaxed, fabric lined plastic gloves being worn alone for wet work together with a liberal powdering of the hands if perspiration is troublesome. Even after all the other local treatment has ceased, a simple emollient cream should be massaged in once or twice a day. This should be continued after gloves are finally abandoned and from this time on the hands should be carefully rinsed in plain water after the wash, and thoroughly and immediately dried. By no account should clothes be hung out to dry with wet hands. Barrier creams have proved disappointing since the best of them are removed by the friction of the wash. Nevertheless, one of the silicon barrier creams may prove helpful as an emollient. Internal treatment plays little part in the control of such dermatitis. Some cases need to be treated in bed and some severe cases need systemic corticosteroids. For itching oral antipruritics, such as sedatives and antihistamines, can be used.

Local Treatment : In an acute case of contact dermatitis the affected part is washed with soap and water, and cleaned with alcohol if the vesicles are ruptured. A wet compressor soaked in 100 per cent solution of tannic acid is applied for 30 minutes. Calomine lotion, hydrocortisone cream/lotion is then applied. Prophylaxis is important in certain contact dermatitis like industrial dermatitis.

Prophylaxis : This applies to industrial dermatitis. One must be careful in selecting workers for various occupations. Usually people with thick, dark, oily skins are, as a rule, less susceptible than those with fair, thin, dry skins. Hairless skin is less likely to be affected by certain industrial lesions. Conditions of work should be cool and perspiration avoided. Ventilation should be sufficient to keep the atmosphere clear of fumes and dust. Special protective clothing such as gloves, mask, goggles, etc., should be issued if necessary. Barrier creams should be available and rubbed in before starting work and after each wash. Barrier creams which protect against various substances are available under various names in the market. Their effect in doing so is often doubtful. Adequate washing facilities should be provided with hot and cold running water and good quality soap. Both management and employees must understand the consequences of dermatitis, and the various measures that can be used to prevent it must be implemented. Desensitisation (hyposensitisation) has not proved possible in a vast majority of examples of contact dermatitis. In the case of penicillin, streptomycin, chlorpromazine, this has been quite successful. Doctors, nurses, dispensers have to continue handling the drugs. The procedure of desensitisation is a prolonged and hazardous one and is done under medical supervision.

Certain conditions also prevail :

1) *Industrial :* Chrome in the form of its acids/salts causes ulcers of skin (chrome holes or chrome ulcers); occupational acne is caused by oil, tar products (industrial acne).

2) *Phyto dermatitis :* Certain plants such as parsnips, hogweed, etc., will produce eruptions if their juice gets on to the skin which is subsequently exposed to the sun.

3) *Purpuic or textile dermatitis :* Chemical substances left on textile material produce purpuric (haemorrhages) papules.

4) *Napkin dermatitis :* This occurs in babies in areas covered by napkins due to soap, soda, detergents left in napkins after washing. This is called Non-Eczematous Dermatitis. These conditions have been mentioned to differentiate and place them in a separate group other than contact dermatitis.

Summary

Three conditions have been discussed in the above section:

a) Urticaria (Hive) can be local or general caused by various factors.

b) Giant urticaria, red urticaria, papular urticaria are various forms of it.

c) Histamine is the main causative agent.

d) Avoiding the various agents causing it is the important aspect in treatment.

2. Allergic Eczema (Atopic type) applies to the person, not to the condition. Family history of allergy is present. Apart from eczema, urticaria or asthma or hay fever is also seen.

   Infantile, puberty, adult are seen. Condition clears on its own.

3. In contact dermatitis various agents by contact produce allergies. Offending agents are to be avoided to get relief.

13

FOOD-DRUG ALLERGIES AND MIGRAINE

Most of the doctors and critics well informed on the subject on allergies may object to the inclusion of migraine in this discussion there are two reasons for including them :

1) As the authors was going through various source materials for collecting information on allergies, they happen to see one particular classification of allergic disorders in which migraine was included. Though it does not have allergic basis, the trigger factors causing an attack of migraine can be compared to allergens causing various reactions. Mechanism may be different but the 'cause-effect' is the basis.

2) Though a 'food allergy' and a 'migraine triggered by an item of food' cannot be equated, a comparison can be made and should not pose a problem to the critics or medicos.

Food Allergies

1) *Food Additives*

Today most of the processed foods contain additives, both natural and man-made. Although consumers have a right to be wary of them, the good news is that most additives are safe and in some cases even beneficial. In fact, more worrisome may be the so-called accidental additives (including pesticides, hormones, antibiotics) that often wind up in our plates. As the demand increased for a year-round supply of many foods, food manufacturers stepped up the use of additives to extend shelf life to ensure the safety and heighten the appeal of their products. Some common categories are:

a) Preservatives : (e.g. anti-oxidants)

b) Fortifiers : Vitamins

c) Colour enhancers : Beta Carotene, FD and C Blue Nos 1 and 2

d) Flavour enhancers : Monosodium glutamate

e) Emulsifiers or thickeners : Gum arabic

f) Humectants : Dextrose, glycerine

There are more than 3,000 approved health additives in various parts of the world. New additives undergo long-term testing before being approved. Food additives like other chemicals may produce effects if consumed in large quantities. However, the quantities in food products are regulated to avert this possibility, except for a very few people, who may be sensitive to certain additives such as sulphites. Adverse reactions are rare.

For the general public, the benefits of additives outweigh the risks. Ironically, the food additives that pose the greatest health risk may be natural, not synthetic: sodium and sugar (often in the form of dextrose, cornsyrup, sucrose, etc.). This increases salt consumption and associated problems. Certain brands of commercial baby foods contain added sugar, salt and modified food starch which is why some health experts recommend organic baby foods. Some research has linked food additives (particularly artificial flavouring, artificial colouring and sugar) with hyperactivity in children. Some additives interact with certain drugs. Possible culprits include nitrites (found in processed meats), cyclamates (artificial sweeteners), methyl polysiloxane (found in cooking oil). Subtracting additives from the diet is an important preventive aspect. One can eat more fresh meat, fish, poultry instead of smoked or processed versions. To limit artificial sweeteners limit the intake of junk food, diet sodas, pre-packaged foods. Opt for fresh foods rather than canned foods. Organic foods are also good options. Natural additives from beets, corn, etc., are not superior to artificial ones.

Food allergy is marked by:

1) Aerophagy (swallowing air or symptoms of gas abdomen)
2) Disturbed appetite
3) Vomiting
4) A loose stool
5) Abdominal pain.

2) *Dairy Foods*

These are the main source of calcium, a nutrient essential to maintaining good health. On the other hand, dairy foods like wholemilk, butter, cream and certain cheeses have large quantities of saturated fat which increase the cholesterol levels and risk of heart disease. But we have reduced fat versions which can be consumed for a healthful diet. It is always better to choose low fat products in dairy food. Milk is a good source of various vitamins, phosphorus, magnesium, protein and calcium of course. About 8 ounces of whole milk provides 20 per cent of the body's daily protein and calcium needs.

All milk sold must be pasteurized. It is not good to drink raw unpasteurised milk on farm visits. Pregnant women and anyone with weakened immune systems should also avoid certain brands of raw milk and cheese as they may trigger allergic reactions due to hypersensitivity. Pasteurized milk may contain small amounts of antibiotics and other drugs. In most of the milks, the levels are

Table 13.1 gives an idea as to what each can do, including allergies, though they are approved in many countries:

Table 13.1 : Food and Their Effects

Additive, Function, Source	*Possible Effects*
a) Aspartame (artificial sweetener) found in soft drinks, chewing gum, in child medications.	may trigger headaches, migraines
b) BHA or BHT (preservative/ antioxidant) in bakery items, potato chips, oils, cereals.	may cause *allergic* reactions
c) FD and C yellow No:5 artificial (tartrazine) colour enhancer found in candy, ice-cream, custards, beverages.	may cause allergic reactions such such as *hives*
d) MSG (monosodium glutamate) considered a food ingredient found in restaurant food, soups, bouillon cubes.	may cause headaches, drowsiness, nausea, rapid head beat, tingling in face or arms
e) Sodium nitrate/sodium nitrite (a preservative, anti-microbial) found in hot dogs, sausages, ham, processed lunch meats, smoked fish.	carcinogenic; interaction with drugs
f) Sorbic acid used as preservative (K Sorbate Ca Sorbate) in yoghurts, pickles, juices, jams, jellies, sauces, processed cheeses.	No adverse effects
g) Sulphites used as a preservative and antioxidant commonly used ones are sodium sulphite, SO_2, Na or K bisulphate Na or K metabi-sulphite) used in dried, canned, frozen fruit; wine; beer, bakery items, precut potatoes, olives botlled lemon juice; maraschino cherries, canned shrimp.	may cause Asthma attacks, hives, diarrhoea, nausea, in some cases *anaphylactic shock*

undetectable or they are so small that they are not deemed harmful. Even pasteurised milk will get spoiled if it is not refrigerated properly.

Cardboard containers are ideal for packing milk as they block out sunlight which can cause vitamin A and riboflavin to breakdown. One should be extremely careful when giving milk to children. Do not give cow's milk to infants under one year of age. It is too high in protein and sodium. For the first six months, bottle-fed babies do not need anything, but infant formula. Low fat milk is not suitable for babies under two years of age. Some young children may be allergic to the protein in cow's milk. Even formula-fed infants may have allergic reactions since many commercial formulas are modified cow's milk. If chronic diarrhoea, vomiting, and colic appear, the doctor must be consulted for diagnosis and suggestions for milk alternatives.

Dairy foods can aggravate ulcers by stimulating production of irritating stomach acid. Aged cheeses can trigger migraines and interact adversely with certain medications. Cheeses made with moulds may trigger penicillin allergies.

One does not have to eliminate milk and milk products when one has a cold or flu. Dairy foods do not promote mucous build-up as many people once thought.

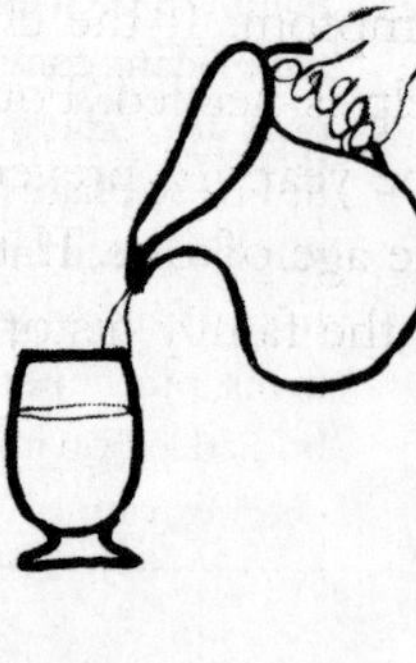

Cheese is nutritious, but is very high in saturated fat. Even reduced fat cheeses contain a high per cent of fat and high Na (sodium). Those with heart disease, high cholesterol, high BP must avoid cheese altogether, or stick to skimmed milk cottage or farmer cheese. Aged cheeses can trigger migraines and cheeses made with moulds can trigger penicillin allergies.

What is lactose intolerance? Milk does not agree with everyone. Difficulty in digesting milk sugar/lactose is believed to be due to decreased levels of the enzyme lactose in stomach. Cramps, diarrhoea, and flatulence are the symptoms. The person must try eating high lactose foods (milk, fresh cheeses, ice-cream) in small amounts as part of meals. He can consume low lactose dairy foods like lactose-reduced milk, yoghurts, etc. If the problem persists, a doctor can do simple tests to find whether lactose intolerance is there or if is it due to other causes lactose supplements are given.

3) *Eggs*

Eggs are nutritious but high in cholesterol. If eaten raw or uncooked they can make one sick. Salmonella, a common bacterium that causes food-borne illness, can be found inside some clean, uncracked eggs; so eating them raw is never safe. Raw eggs are to be avoided in home-made preparations like mayonnaise or ice-cream. Liquid, pasteurized egg products, free of cholesterol and salmonella, can now be found in some supermarkets. Eggs can cause allergic reactions in children under the age of three. Itchy hives on skin usually around the mouth are a common symptom. If the child has breathing trouble, immediate medical help is needed. For most children, egg allergies disappear within one year. To prevent them, avoid giving egg to an infant before the age of one. If the baby is being breastfed and there is allergy in the family history, eggs must be avoided for the duration.

4) *Nuts and Seeds*

Prepared nuts and nut butters are often made with cholesterol raising trans fats and saturated fats that undermine their healthfulness. Nuts have high calorie and fat counts. They are among the most common potentially dangerous food allergens. Nuts include tree nuts (pecans, almonds), seeds (sunflower, pumpkin) and some legumes including the misleadingly named peanut. All contain high percentage of fat calories (50 to 75 per cent of total calories). Brazie nuts, pine nuts, macadamias contain very high percentage of saturated fat. The fats in other nuts are mainly mono and polysaturated. Peanuts contain antioxidants which protect against heart disease. All nuts decrease LDL or bad cholesterol in our blood and protect against heart attacks. Nuts are also inhibitors of cancer cell growth. They contain omega 3 fatty acids (almonds, walnuts, flaxseeds are very good sources of omega 3FA) which decrease the risk of clots and stroke. Nuts are good sources of proteins, vitamins, and minerals. Salted peanuts which are used as snacks are very high in salt content. Peanut butters may have high percentage of partially hydrogenated oils. These two should be limited. Nuts and peanuts can trigger fatal reactions in people allergic to them. But avoiding them can be tough.

1) Read labels carefully. Peanut oils and butters, groundnuts and other nut products are used by processors to prepare anything and everything from chilli and sauces to ice-creams and candy bars.

2) Stay away from many of the Asian and Middle Eastern cuisines in which nuts are common ingredients. This 'allergy allert' is for nut sensitive individuals.

3) If you eat out review the menu with the chef to make certain the foods are safe for you and the seriousness of your allergy is understood.

The above three precautions taken can help sensitive persons prevent the allergic reactions triggered by nuts.

Washing away Allergens

Peanut allergy is the third most common allergy in young children and the most common in older kids, teens and adults. There have been considerable discussions on how best to protect allergic people from inadvertent exposure to peanuts. Soap-free hand sanitisers apparently are not enough. Researchers from Johns Hopkins' Children Centre in Baltimore applied a teaspoon of peanut butter to the hands of 19 non-allergic adults and then had them wash their hands with a variety of cleansers, plain water and an alcohol-based hand sanitiser. Hand wipes, liquid soap and bar soap removed all of the allergens that sets off allergic reactions. Water and the hand sanitiser left some behind.

The study appeared in the May 2004 issue of the *Journal of Allergy and Clinical Immunology.*

5) *Fruits and Vegetables*

Fruits are good sources of flavinoids as well as fibre, vitamins and minerals. Vegetables are rich in fibres and vitamins, and also have right proportions of the minerals sodium and potassium. They also have good quantities of folate or folic acid.

Both fruits and vegetables offer benefits in terms of (1) anti-cancer effects (2) balancing BP (3) prevention of stroke (4) decreased risk of coronary heart disease. Flavinoids in fruits act as antioxidants and prevent cancers. Apples, apricots, bananas, oranges, papayas, plums, watermelons, grapes, dates, figs are high sources of vitamin C, vitamin A and fibres. Tomatoes provides lycopenes, sprouts are rich sources proteins, carrots and other raw vegetables provide caronoids and other nutrients.

But certain sensitive individuals can develop allergies with fruits and vegetables. Allergy to citrus fruits like oranges, grape fruit, lemons have been noted in sensitive individuals. Tomatoes, onions, potatoes, cauliflower, brinjal, etc., have been known to produce allergies. Dried fruits and some canned, bottled, frozen or glazed fruits often contain sulphites which preserve colour but can trigger severe asthma attacks, even anaphylactic shock, in susceptible people. Pre-packaged products containing sulphites must state this on the label. Products purchased in bins are exempt however. If a person is susceptible, he should check the package label to be sure that fruits contain no sulphites.

Pesticide residues can also trigger allergies. The exposure can be reduced by rinsing and peeling the fruit/vegetable or by choosing organic fruits. Microbacterial contaminations must also be kept in mind. Scrub the fruit under cold water with a brush to avoid various contaminations. In sensitive individuals, the culprit fruit or vegetable must be avoided to prevent allergic reactions.

6) *Shellfishes, Salad Bars*

Shellfishes are rich in protein, omega 3 fatty acids, calcium, zinc, iron, vitamin B and right amounts of cholesterol (it is not high as it was once thought). Among shellfishes, oysters, mussels and crabs contain omega 3 fatty acids in high levels which control high BP, cholesterol, etc., have a cardio-protective role. Shellfishes can absorb contaminants from the sea and can cause allergic reactions in sensitive individuals. Cooking them thoroughly can reduce the bacterial contamination. They may absorb pollutants and toxins if they live in contaminated water. They should be avoided. Anyone at risk for 'gout' should avoid foods rich in uric acid such as shellfishes.

Salad bars offer salads with a variety of greens, vegetables, fruits, beans, seeds, meat. It is very important to know what is in your salad before you buy it from a salad bar or hotel. For a healthful salad, it should be a simple one. The darkest greens like spinach, vegetables like broccoli, carrots, peas or fresh fruits like oranges, apples, melons kidney beans, small pieces of lean meat and modest amount of light dressing (if any at all) all these make up a health salad. Sulphites, preservatives once commonly added to cut fruits and vegetables to keep them looking fresh were banned (for this use) because of their potential to trigger severe allergic reactions, but salad bars offer many other items such as macaroni, cheese, fried chicken wings, creamy soups, etc. They are near the salads and contamination can trigger allergies in sensitive individuals. Sometimes one particular ingredient of salad (either a vegetable bean or fruit) may trigger allergy. Therefore, the sensitive individual should first check the contents of salad to verify that it does not contain any offending ingredient or he can order a 'salad' in such a way that it contains only ingredients that agree with him.

7) *Wheat Allergy*

We have already mentioned about this in factors causing asthma. Gluten-sensitive enteropathies are common manifestations of wheat allergy. Gluten and the derivative gliadin are proteins found in wheat, barley, rye and grains. A hypersensitivity reaction to antigenic components within gliadin causes intestinal changes like loss of food absorbing villi in the small intenstine. It is usually common in children. Antigenic challenge by gliadin leads to synthesis of antibodies in the intestine. Faulty absorption, muscle cramps, anemia, etc., are observed. Like milk, wheat also produces allergy in infants (due to cereal) and can produce gastro intestine symptoms, rashes, etc. Avoidance of wheat is suggested.

A few points for noting are:

1) there can be cross-reaction between various seafoods. Those allergic to fish must avoid other seafoods also.

2) Persons allergic to nuts must avoid preparations like cakes and cookies which contain nuts.

3) Chocolates can cause allergies either as plain chocolates or in combination with milk and nuts added to make tasty chocolate bars.

4) Soft drinks and mushrooms also can produce allergies.

Treatment begins after a complete history and symptoms of allergy (hives, urticaria, even anaphylaxis) are studied. Skin tests can be done; eliminating the culprit in diet is often shown to bring relief from allergic symptoms. Desensitisation to foods is not done usually. Cooked foods are prescribed in the place of raw foods in many cases as being *de natured* they are less allergenic.

Drug Allergy

We have already discussed about 'dermatitis medicamentosa', a condition in contact dermatitis which is due to the external application of a medicament. Drug eruptions are defined as any cutaneous abnormality caused by ingestion, inhalation or injection of a medicament. The pathology mechanism of drug eruptions is obscure and varies from one drug to the next. Sometimes it is an allergic response as in the case of penicillin. Other drugs, for instance, heavy metals, cause toxic reactions like purpura (bleeding) and exfoliative dermatitis. Some individuals appear to have an 'inherent idiosyncrasy' reacting to small doses with peculiar lesions which cannot be reproduced in the majority of individuals.

In the majority of cases, however, the causative mechanism has still to be elucidated. Drugs may cause practically every known type of cutaneous lesion varying from single, small and localised plaques like 'fixed drug eruption' caused by phenolphthalein to universal and fatal exfoliative dermatitis due to gold or arsenic. The reaction may follow within a few hours of taking the drug as in the case of penicillin or aspirin or may be delayed for months (anti-malarials) or years (arsenic). Fever is a common accompaniment; involvement of buccal mucosa and enlargement of lymph glands are also seen. Sometimes other tissues and organs may also be involved leading to various blood dyscarsias, hepatitis, nephritis (inflammation in liver, kidney) etc. Diagnosis depends mostly on the constant awareness of the possibility of a drug eruption.

Occult sources such as suppositories and pessaries should be sought by careful questioning. The typical acute eruption occurs from one to 24 hours after the last dose and is sudden in onset. It is usually widespread and affects especially the trunks and proximal parts of the limbs, bright in colour and symmetrical. It subsides promptly on withdrawing the causative drug. The morphology of the eruption may point to the responsible 'drug' since most drugs have a limited repertoire. However, any drug is capable of producing on occasion any eruption. The final diagnosis depends on the result of stopping the suspected substance. Patch tests, as has been emphasised, are not applicable, and intradermal tests are of no value. Positive proof can be got only by giving a small dose of the drug by mouth, a practice which is fraught with danger and should never be undertaken.

In spite of the enormous increase in consumption of drugs, drug eruptions are surprisingly infrequent and there are relatively few common cases. The commonest are those due to sedatives, hypnotics especially the barbiturates. Second come antibiotics and chemotherapeutic agents, particularly penicillin, streptomycin and sulphonamides. Other drugs, important because of their frequency of use of severity of reaction, are aspirin, codeine, phenylbutazone, heavy metals, antisera. Some of the important eruptions caused by these and other drugs will be described in more detail.

1) *Erythema (Reddening)*

This is the commonest of drug reactions and this may be in the confluent, patchy, macular or scarlatina form. It is most frequently due to barbiturates. Other hypnotics are chloral, chlorpromazine, sulphonamides, streptomycin. It is rapidly reversible on stopping the drug. There may be fever and this also subsides with the rashes.

2) *Urticaria*

This is also very common and is particularly due to penicillin, aspirin and antisera. In the case of antisera, it may be severe and widespread and accompanied by fever, headache, general malaise, pains in joints, albumenuria (albumin in urine), and nephritis. Two other peculiarities of penicillin urticaria are that its onset may be delayed for as long as one month after the last dose and that once it has begun, it can continue for months or years after discontinuing the drug. The mechanism of these two phenomena remains obscure. Occasionally continuing urticaria may be traced to small amounts of penicillin in milk or in the hospital wards or to other occult sources such as vaccines but usually no cause can be found. Aspirin is an extremely common constituent of proprietary medicaments such as are widely advertised in the lay press and sold from all types of shops and even slot machines (in Western countries). Exhaustive questioning may therefore be necessary in investigating the case of urticaria suspected of being a drug eruption. Griseofulvin (an antifungal medicine) is another, though much less, common cause.

3) *Purpura* (*Bleeding in Skin*)

This may occur in very severe erythematous or urticarial reactions and represents no more than the ultimate in vaso dilatation (expansion of blood vessels). Eruptions due to anti-coagulants, such as phenindione, begin as erythematous but later become purpuric. (In Erythema redness is obturated by pressure but not in purpura. This is an important difference.) Drugs like carbromal produce toxic effect on skin blood vessels. This leads to a patchy, purpuric eruption (which is pigmented and scaly) on the skin. Drugs like phenylbutazone, chlorothiazide (a diuretic) and meprobamate also produce purpuric lesions on skin.

4) *Bulbous Eruption (Small to Big Blisters filled with Serum)*

These are produced by barbiturates and sulphonamides. Even after the drug is withdrawn, the eruptions persist.

5) *Anceiform Eruptions*

These are caused by iodides, bromides and anti-convulsants like Tridione. The lesions are papular and pustular and occur in the face, neck and shoulders. Steroids can also produce such lesions. Sometimes lesions caused by iodide and bromide become large, fungating seen on the face and limbs.

6) *Lichenoid (Shiny, Flat-topped Papules)*

These are caused by anti-malarials, arsenicals, gold, phenothaizines, PAS, chlorothiazide, etc.

7) *Exfoliative Dermatitis*

This is a serious condition in which the whole of the skin becomes red, thickened and scaly. It can prove fatal. Any drug eruption which is very serious can evolve into this condition if it is very severe or if the drug is continued after the original eruption has begun. Certain drugs like arsenicals, gold, mercury, sulphonamides, and streptomycin can produce this as a primary reaction.

8) *Light Sensitivity Eruptions*

These are caused by sulphonamides, chlorpromazine (largactil), antibiotics and chlorothiazide. Erythematous lesions or eczematous lesions are seen as slate blue/grey pigmentation of skin, especially of the face. This is seen in patients with long time continued high doses of largactil. Along with this are seen granular deposits on cornea and vision. Vision impairment can occur.

9) *Fixed Drug Eruption*

One or more well defined circular patches of dusky redness (erythema) appear on trunk or proximal portion of limbs a few hours after taking the drug, and can last for two-three days. The lesions can be bulbous and affected areas may develop pigmentation. Phenotphthalin (present in laxatives), cause this lesion.

10) *Arsenic*

Prolonged ingestion of inorganic arsenic such as used to be given for psoriasis and dermatitis herpetiformis and added to bromides for epilepsy and iron for anemia can cause cutaneous change many years after the patient has ceased taking the drug.

Such cases are therefore still seen and show multiple small warty excrescences known as Punctate Keratoses in palms, soles, trunk, limbs. Pigmentation called 'Raindrop pigmentation' is seen on the trunk. The skin may also show epitheliomata carcinomata as is seen in bronchus. Liver cirrhosis is also a sequel cross sensitisation phenomenon. Some patients develop a sensitivity to more than one drug; this can be explained by the fact that they react to a 'particular chemical group' present in a number of chemically-related compounds. For example, in 'para aminophenol group' seen in sulphonamides, 'benzocaine group' of anaesthetics; patients can react to such substances throughout their lives. Care is to be taken to avoid giving other drugs of this group to a sensitive individual as all of them will have the particular chemical unit in them. Generally, a patient sensitive to one penicillin will be reacting to all since the sensitivity is to the "penicillin nucleus" which is common to all types.

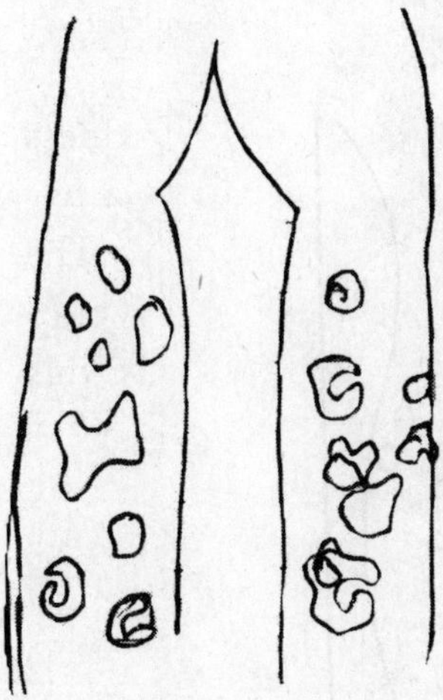

Fig. 13.1 : Fungating Papillmaous Type Bromide Eruptions

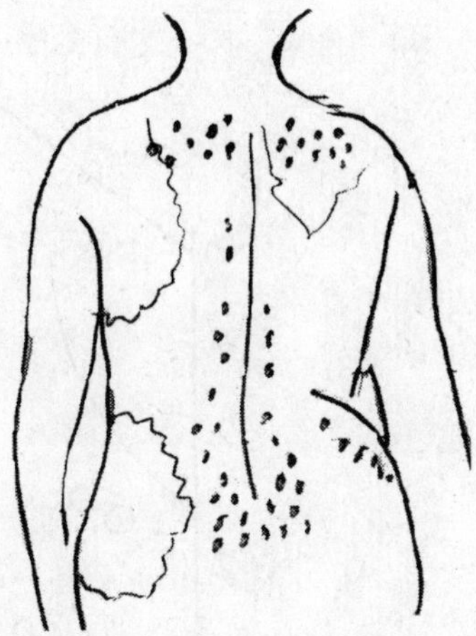

Fig. 13.2 : Gold Dermatitis

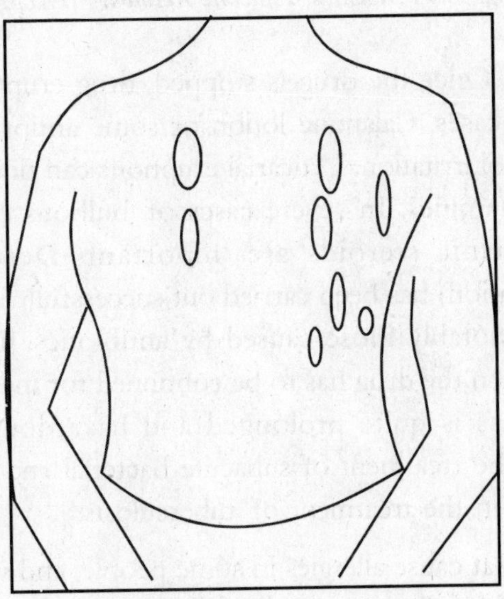

Fig. 13.3 : Arsenical (Raindrop) Pigmentation

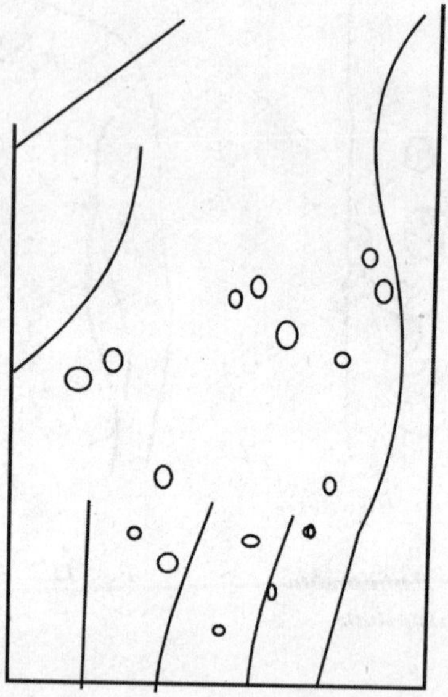

Fig. 13.4 : Arsenical Punctate Keratoses (PALM)

Treatment : Once the drug is stopped, drug eruptions clear in most of the cases. Calamine lotion or some antipruritic can be used to control irritation. Urticarial eruptions can find some relief with anti-histamines. In severe cases of bulbous or exfoliative lesions systemic steroids are important. Desensitisation (hyposensitisation) has been carried out successfully in some drug sensitivities, notably those caused by antibiotics. This is to be done only when the drug has to be continued for medical reasons as the process is quite prolonged and hazardous. Example: Penicillin in the treatment of subacute bacterial endocarditis and streptomycin in the treatment of tuberculosis.

some drugs that cause allergies in some people, and which special mention are the following are the following:

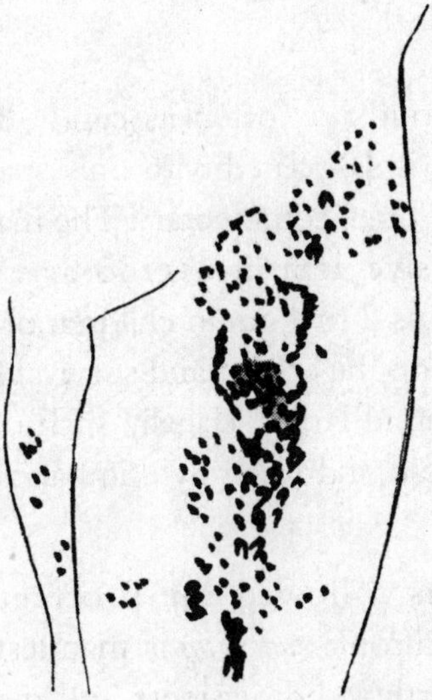

Fig. 13.5 : Carbromal Drug Eruption

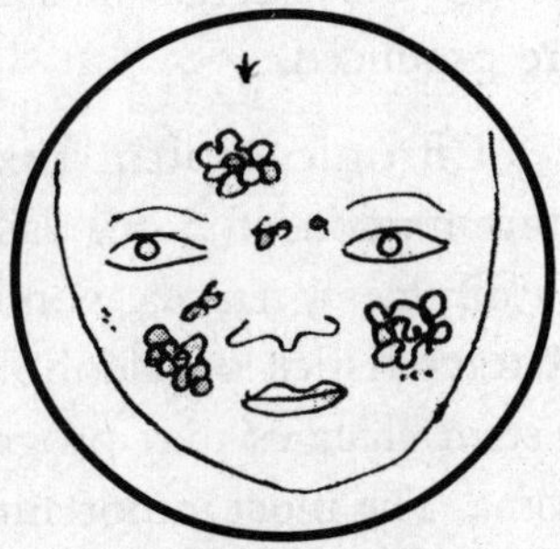

Fig. 13.6 : Fungating Type

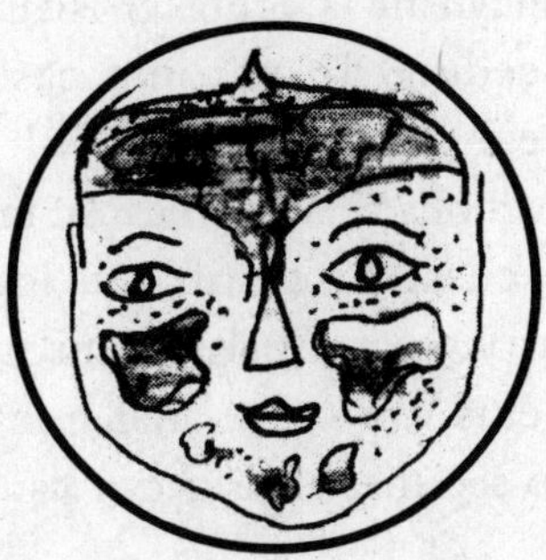

Fig. 13.7 : Sulphonamide Dermatitis

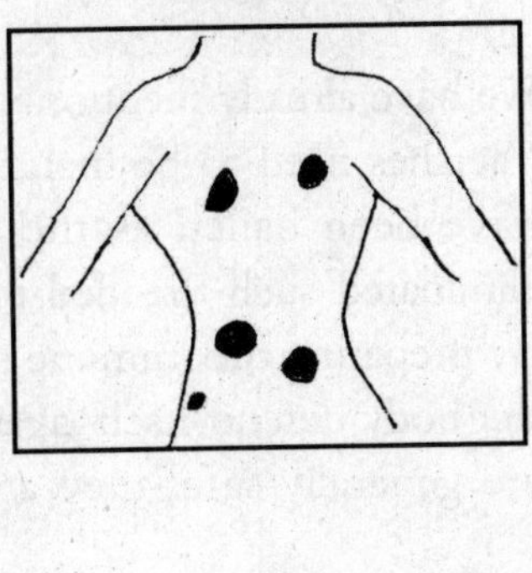

Fig. 13.8 : Fixed Drup Eruption

1. *Aspirin (Acetyl Salicylic Acid)*

Despite its being popped into mouths as often as candy, and despite its potential toxicity aspirin is associated with only sparse morphologic changes meriting only brief commentary. The major untoward consequences of massive aspirin overdosage are metabolic. The ingestion of as little as 2 to 4 gm in children or 10 to 30 gm in adults may be fatal but on the other hand survival has been reported following doses fivefold larger. Usually such over dosage is accidental or suicidal. Fluid and electrolyte imbalances are produced.

Chronic aspirin toxicity has followed the protracted consumption of 3 gm daily. This chronic *salicylism* is manifested by dizziness, nausea, vomiting, diarrhoea, drowsiness and many characteristics of alcoholic intoxication. The central nervous system changes may progress to hallucinations, convulsions and coma. The most important morphologic consequence of chronic salicylism is acute erosive gastritis leading to gastro-intestinal bleeding. In chronic cases important chemicals in clotting mechanisms leads to bleeding. Sometimes hypersensitivity reactions to aspirin cause urticaria, multiform skin rashes (already discussed), exfoliative dermatitis, acute asthmatic attacks, anaphylaxis. Analgesic mixtures of aspirin and phenactein or other agents can cause analgesic nephropathy (kidney damage). Thus we see that aspirin can cause serious allergic reactions.

2. *Vaccines*

We have already mentioned about antiserum-induced skin rashes. Vaccines need to be mentioned in detail. We know that vaccines have been hailed as the medical miracles and have virtually eliminated such dreaded illnesses as smallpox, polio, diphtheria. By preparing the immune system to fight off infection, they help the body defend itself against certain diseases. Though vaccines are generally safe, they are not risk- free, and there are some important cautions to note. They can cause mild side effects including redness or pain at the site of injection, fatigue, sore muscles and fever. If a person is allergic to eggs or baker's yeast, he must inform the doctor. In rare cases, there may be an allergic reaction to the vaccine itself, the materials in which it was grown, or the chemicals in which it was suspended. For example, if a person has egg allergy, he must be beware of flue shots or the MMR vaccine. Since both are grown in egg medium, people who are allergic to the drug neomycin are urged to avoid the chickenpox vaccine available in USA, but not yet licensed in Canada. Thus we see that every country has its own reservations and specifications.

DTP vaccine was linked to sudden infant death syndrome, brain damage, etc., but there were no conclusive evidence regarding this doubt. Finally, vaccines are not 100 per cent fail-safe (though they are often close). One reason is that a person's immune system may not respond to a vaccine as it should. Certain vaccines and their potential risks are given below:

	Risks Include
a) DTP Vaccine (Diphtheria Tetanus pertussis)	Very small chances of seizures, severe allergic reaction (or) brain damage. Children who should not get pertussis vaccine should get Td vaccine, not DTP.
b) Polio	OPV—Very small chance of getting polio, IPV—no risk.
c) MMR	Could trigger an allergic reaction to eggs or drug neomycin. May cause fall in blood platelets.
d) Hepatitis B	Extremely small chances of serious allergic reaction or anaphylactic shock.

e)	Hib (Heaemophilus influenza type B)	Very small chance of getting paralytic polio.
f)	Influenza vaccine	Could trigger an allergic reaction to eggs. There is an extremely small risk of a severe paralytic illness.

3) *Penicillin*:

In remarkably safe drug, the only important reaction to be feared is anaphylaxis. Intolerance is a major problem with penicillin therapy and includes idiosyncratic, anaphylactic and allergic reactions. The risk of reactions is 5 to 10 per cent with benzathine penicillin, 2 to 5 per cent with procaine penicillin and 1 to 3 per cent with benzyne penicillin. When these are administered by injections, the mortality in severe reactions has been assessed at 9 to 13 per cent. The incidence of these reactions is considered to be very high when benzylpenicillin is used either topically or in aerosol form, and it appears to be least when the drug is taken orally. However, fatalities have occurred following ingestion of penicillin. Some individuals are so sensitive that the mere handling of a tablet of penicillin or just a skin test dose may cause immediate severe reaction in them. Further, severe reactions have been recorded following the first dose of penicillin in persons who had never received the drug before. This is probably because of the fact that many of us are exposed and slightly sensitised to various common airborne moulds that readily grow on and elaborate— penicillin and penicillin-like substances in foodstuffs such as bread, fruit, oil with or without decay. Penicillin sensitisation can also occur from the presence of the drug in the environment of patients using penicillin aerosols and by ingesting milk containing penicillin. The present evidence indicates that the commercial penicillin may contain powerful proteinaceous antigen with penicilloyl specificity which can cause severe reactions in sensitive people. Since modification of penicillin may remove the protecinaceous residue some of the semi-synthetic penicillins may be less dangerous in this respect. Alimentary digestion of this material may explain the smaller incidence of anaphylaxis on oral administration of such preparations. The semi synthetic penicillins are however cross-allergenic in varying degrees with the natural penicillin.

The important allergic manifestations are :

a) *Skin rashes of various types* : We have already discussed this. These are associated with itching and these 'rash plus itching' are the most common of the allergic reactions. These may appear at any time during penicillin therapy or even one to two weeks after discontinuation of treatment. Severe reactions like exfoliative dermatitis are however rare.

b) *A serum sickness-like syndrome* : This is characterised by rash, fever, increased eosonophil count (eosonophilia), lymphadenopathy, angioneurotic oedema, asthma, arthralgia and may appear seven to 10 days after penicillin therapy. In some cases, purpura, myocarditis, hematuria (blood in urine) develop. Sometimes only fever with or without increased eosonophil count is the only manifestation. It usually subsides two to three days after the discontinuation of the treatment.

c) *Renal disturbances like hematuria and albuminuria* (blood and albumin in urine) : These are rare.

d) *Hemopoietic disturbances like hemolytic anemia* (increased breakdown of RBC and haemoglobin level goes down): These occur very rarely. The patients show serum antibodies against penicillin.

e) *Anaphylaxis* : This is the most serious reaction but occurs in fewer than 0.1 per cent of patients. The symptoms of anaphylaxis begins within few minutes after penicillin administration. Anaphylaxis can develop with minute quantities of penicillin and irrespective of route or administration. It is characterised by an acute cardiovascular collapse, broncho spasm, angioedema, particularly oedema of the larynx. It is believed that penicilloic acid, either alone or linked to a plasma protein, is responsible for these reactions.

Tests for detection of penicillin allergy : No reliable method. History of allergy and positive skin test are all not complete evidence of allergy *nor* does a negative history or negative skin test indicate the safety of penicillin administration.

Skin Tests : One method of skin testing is to scratch the skin through a drop of solution containing 10,000 units of benzyl penicillin/ml. If a central wheal due to local oedema occurs after 15 minutes, it is considered a positive reaction. These are not very reliable. Persons with negative skin test may get fatal anaphylaxis with the drug, and positive skin test persons may tolerate penicillin without allergic reactions. Also the small test of penicillin dose used for a skin test may itself produce severe reaction.

Another skin test involves administration of 0.05 ml of penicilloyl-polylysine intradermally and subsequent observation of inflammatory response. This test is often combined with benzyne penicillin scratch test. A combination of these two tests is considered to predict virtually all reactions to penicillin. Scratch test should precede the intradermal test to avoid any dangerous reaction following the latter. Serological methods to detect specific antibodies, etc., are difficult, costly, unreliable. Penicillin antibodies are easily detected but are present even in normal subjects without history of allergy. There is hence no value for such tests.

If a person with a positive skin test has to be administered penicillin for a life-threatening infection, penicillin desensitisation should be carried out under cover of corticosteroid and anti-histaminic therapy (as already mentioned). Benzyl penicillin in the dose of 500 units should be administered initially, and the dose is increased gradually till therapeutic levels are reached. Further, cortiocosteroids may have to be administered in very large doses (50-100 mg of prednisolone per day) to prevent the development of anaphylaxis. Such large doses of steroids may affect the host resistance, and this must be weighed against the beneficial anti- allergic effect desired. Serum bactericidal tests should be performed to evaluate and monitor the bactericidal regimen employed, since the clinical picture of the disease may be altered by steroids. Anti-histamines do not decrease the incidence of anaphylaxis. They are however, valuable in controlling the commonly occurring minor allergic reactions.

Apart from the allergic reactions mentioned for penicillin, penicillin treatment can cause other allergic reactions mentioned for penicillin like super infections, hyperkalaemia, acute non-allergic reactions, certain anxiety states, mental disturbances etc. (all these are seen only in *prolonged* administration of benzyl penicillin).

Migraine

A booklet published from Kochi for the Malayala Manorama Co. Ltd. includes migraine (sick headache) in its common allergic diseases list. Migraine is triggered by many common allergy-causing substances like 'food substances' which are very important precipitating factors in migraine.

What is Migraine ?

Migraine is the name given to a particular pattern of recurring physical symptoms of which the most distressing is usually the headache. These symptoms vary in their nature and in the severity and frequency in sufferers. In most cases, it is very easy to decide if some one has migraine but occasionally there is uncertainty because the diagnosis is made purely on the symptoms. Despite the ever increasing complexity of tests available in medicine, today there is still no test for migraine. It is of course essential that the correct diagnosis is made, otherwise there can be no rational treatment. Most of the symptoms of migraine are non-specific, that is, they also occur in other conditions. Headache occurs in nearly 50 different medical disorders, some of which are serious but the vast majority are not. All headache sufferers wonder at some time whether they have a brain tumour. This is almost invariably not the case, and with increasing knowledge of headache, it is now possible to decide whether the headache is due to migraine, tension headache or some other condition.

In numerical terms, two disorders account for most headaches: muscle contraction headache (tension) and migraine. A third type cluster headache is also prevalent. This condition is often confused with migraine. The symptoms of migraine have been recognised for over 2,000 years and many famous people have suffered from it—Charles Darwin, Frederic Chopin, Virginia Woolf and David Frost to name but a few, but only in the past 50 years we have had some clues as to its nature and developed effective treatments. The basic cause of the disease is still unclear.

The word migraine comes from a Greek term for a one-sided headache (hemi-orain-ia), but migraine does not have to be one-sided nor are all one-sided headaches due to migraine. Migraine always includes other symptoms alongwith headache. There can be neurological symptoms; sickness is very common and can sometimes be the worst feature of the attack. Hence the name 'sick headache'.

The physical symptoms of migraine are:

a) *Headache* : The worst part of the migraine attack is headache. It is one-sided in nearly 70 per cent cases. The pain builds up slowly over minutes or hours, and becomes severe. Pain is always subjective and difficult to quantify. The duration of headache is usually within the range of a few hours to three days. Head movements, straining, walking can worsen the headache. Sites of headaches change in different attacks, and the pain may be throbbing or stabbing in nature.

b) *Sickness* : As mentioned earlier the 'sickness' complaint has been given the name 'sick headache' to migraine. Ninety-five per cent of migraine attacks are associated with nausea.

There may be vomiting in some cases. Sometimes vomiting relieves headache.

c) *Photophobia and Phonophobia* : These are dislike of light and sound, both of which can occur in a migraine attacks.

d) *Osmophobia* : The dislike of smells such as cooking smells or perfume occurs in many sufferers during migraine attacks.

Changes in temperature, sensation, changes in bowel habits, changes in urinary frequency and changes in blood vessels can also occur during migraine attack.

Various (1) neurological symptoms (aura of migraine) (2) visual symptoms (scintillating scotoma, shimmering lights, fortification spectrum, etc.)., (3) pins and needles sensation on limbs, (4) affected speech (5) alterations in consciousness, double vision, dizziness, etc., can all happen in migraine attacks.

Varieties of Migraine

a) *Common Migraine* : There is one-sided headache, nausea, photo and phonophobias. This is stimulated or triggered by events, circumstances, sensory stimuli and food. All these are called 'Trigger Factors'. The popular terms such as dietary, weekend, menstrual and foot ballers migraine are all synonymous with common migraine.

b) *Classical Migraine* : Here the attacks are preceded by neurological symptoms (called as Aura). Many varieties of classical migraine exist like Vertebro Basilar Migraine, Retinal Migraine, etc.

Children usually have higher incidence of common migraine and not other types. They may suffer from a migraine equivalent called Abdominal Migraine which is recurrent attacks of severe, prolonged stomach pain associated with nausea, vomiting, etc. These symptoms are thought to be related to migraine. Some children go onto have more typical migraine in later life.

Headaches other than migraine are (1) tension (muscle contraction) headaches, (2) cluster headaches (a serious of headaches occur in clusters), (3) secondary headaches like neuralgias, facial pain, ear and eye-pain related headaches etc.

A knowledge of these headaches and their symptoms, etc., helps one in differentiating it from migraine headache. Just as alcohol can cause a headache, so too can monosodium glutamate (Chinese restaurant syndrome), nitrites and nitrates (hot dog headache).

Chinese Restaurant Headache : Chinese meals contain a lot of monosodium glutamate (a substance that enhances flavouring). Some people find that within half hour of starting a Chinese meal (particularly soup) they develop a headache which is usually in the forehead and temples. Besides the headache they may experience pressure or tightness over the face and chest.

Hot Dog Headache : Nitrites are used in curing meat to give it a uniform colour. These substances are also vasodilators (dilate the blood vessels) so that some people find that soon after eating these meats, they develop flushing of the face and a headache. The hot dog is the classical example, but other culprits include ham, bacon, salami.

Withdrawal of caffeine, ergotamine, analgesics can all cause headaches.

Cough, exertion, high BP, etc. can also cause headaches.

Ice-Cream Headache : If a cold substance such as ice-cream or an iced cold drink is swallowed or held in the mouth, the intense cooling causes headache. This is more common in migraine susceptible individuals. The headache is in the frontal region, but in migraine-patients it is in the habitual site of the migraine headache. Such headaches may result from diving in cold water also.

Once we have the knowledge of these headaches, we can avoid the confusion in diagnosis of migraine. Diagnosis of migraine is done by taking a history of symptoms and trying a specific form of therapy.

Tests for Migraine

a) *The Cytotoxic Test* : Foods are often blamed as the cause of migraine and it appears that alcohol, chocolate, cheese, citrus fruit can trigger migraine in some people although we do not know how these foods set off the attack. If a blood sample is taken from a migraine sufferer and small amounts are added to extracts of various foods then some of the blood cells may be damaged by the food extracts. This damage can be seen through a microscope and so on testing against a number of food extracts, a profile of so called food allergies can be determined. This is the principle of the test and it is attractive but it is of no proven use in the management of migraine. The results of the test depends on lab doing the test. Medical literature concludes that it is an unreliable test in terms of validity and reproducibility. It is also an expensive test. However, if a food substance is going to produce migraine, it should do so within 24 hours of consumption, and the cause should usually be obvious.

b) *Skin Tests* : Food extracts are injected into the skin. After a while any reaction produced in the skin is noted and it is then inferred that, that food extract can cause migraine in that patient. There is a clearer association between this test and allergic conditions like asthma, where this sort of test is useful. Most of the medical world says and agrees that migraine is *not* an allergic condition and hence the skin test and migraine have no correlation.

c) *Radio Absorbent Test :* This measures antibodies in the blood to certain foods. Since there is *no* correlation between antibodies and migraine, this test is of *no* use in predicting the cause of migraine. There is only one way of finding out the triggers of migraine and that is by looking for patterns of association.

Blood tests, x-ray, lumbar puncture, EEG, brain scan, angiography—these diagnostic investigations are done in other types of headaches like the ones associated with temporal arteritis, headaches associated with teeth, neck, sinus, pituitary problems, meningitis, SA haemorrhage and headaches associated with skull lesions.

Pathogenesis of Migraine: There is a common mechanism to the production of migraine. The nature of this reaction or long pathway is still controversial. It is not a disease in the usual meaning of the word since, while it causes much suffering, it produces no long term physical or mental disability. The only common finding among sufferers during an attack is the desire to withdraw from the world to seek out a dark, quiet stimulus- free environment where sleep will bring out recovery. If migraine does serve any purpose it may be the removal of the sufferer from the triggers of migraine. In many sufferers, this possible defence mechanism appears to be very active. One day it may be possible to describe the process of migraine in clear biochemical terms and explain how it can be triggered. We are still a long way from this goal.

The cause of migraine is multifactorial and depends both on (1) the genetic make up the individual, i.e., inherent personality traits and (2) factors in the environment.

Migraine is a very common condition; 10 per cent of men and 20 per cent of women according to one estimate suffer from migraine at some time in their lives. Migraine improves with age. Comparatively children (boy > girls) are more affected than old people. Migraine has been shown to be a strongly inherited condition—about 70 per cent sufferers have a close family member with the condition.

Except for hemiphlegic migraine (a type of classical migraine) which can affect most of the family starting at a similar age, having common trigger factors, all the other migraines show no close correlations in trigger factors, etc., as far as inheritance is concerned.

Migraine may start first at any age but it is unusual to start after the age of 50. It is evenly distributed throughout the social strata. Many people with migraine show signs of anxiety and depression. Whether this is the cause or the result of migraine is to be debated.

Migraine is a recurring condition in which the periods between attacks are without any symptoms. Attacks may be set off in a variety of ways by what are collectively called trigger factors. Trigger factors can be environmental. This is divided into:

a) Internal—cyclical events like sleep or menstruation which are within us.

b) External—the circumstances or situations found during daily life including various sensory and other stimuli to which we are constantly exposed.

Among the internal factors sleep and menstruation can trigger migraine attacks. Associated with menstruation we can include pregnancy, menopause, hormone replacement treatment, the pill, etc., to influence migraine.

Among the external factors are stress precipitates migraine, bright light, loud noise, strong smells (triggers migraine), hot humid climate, stormy weather (precipitates migraine), food as a migraine trigger is a controversial area.

Books have been written claiming that the right diet can cure migraine, but this is not strictly true. There is no cure for migraine as it is a result of the effect of environmental factors upon predisposed individuals. Some attacks can be avoided but there is no guaranteed cure. Of course everyone wants to find a tangible cause for attacks with the hope that by avoiding the cause, they will no longer get migraine and there is no more tangible substance than food. Furthermore food allergy is fashionable and more respectable than admitting to symptoms of anxiety, stress, depression. A wide variety of foods may set off migraine. Food probably accounts for about 10 per cent of migraine attacks. Scientific proof is very little in this fact. The most commonly implicated food factors are alcohol, chocolate, cheese, citrus fruits. The quantity of each required to prevent an attack appears to vary considerably from person to person.

Experiments have shown that red wine triggers migraine in some people usually within 12 hours of consumption. Port and fortified wines may act generally. Alcohol even in small quantities can trigger an attack. Chocolate is the next commonly proclaimed provoking factor. Scientific trials are on to investigate the evidence that chocolate causes migraine. Cheese, particularly strong cheese, appears to be a trigger. In some, dairy products in general set off attacks. Fruits like oranges, lemons, grapes also trigger attacks. Not only are the fresh fruits important, but also soft drinks and flavourings based on them. Other foods mentioned as trigger factors include nuts, pork, tomatoes, fried foods, wheat. Missing meals can also be a trigger factor for migraine attacks. Migraines triggered by different factors are known by different names like:

Weekened Migraine, Dietary Precipitated Migraine, and Menstrual Migraine. The condition is the same, only the factors are different.

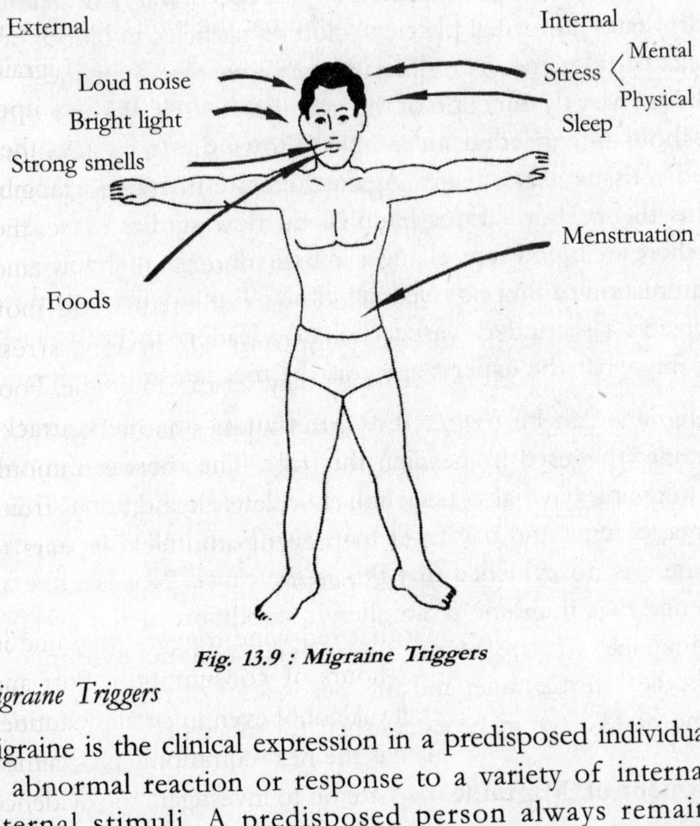

Fig. 13.9 : Migraine Triggers

Migraine Triggers

Migraine is the clinical expression in a predisposed individual of an abnormal reaction or response to a variety of internal or external stimuli. A predisposed person always remains a predisposed person but the clinical expression can change and be changed. Migraine is thus *not a* disease in the usual meaning of the word.

Trigger factors have to reach a certain threshold-stimulus before they can set off an attack. Usually attacks occur by a combination of various trigger factors. The concept of summation of trigger factors is based purely on clinical experience. 'Vascular theory' and 'Neural theory' try to explain the changes which occur in a migraine attack. 'Aura is due to the constriction of arteries supplying blood to brain and subsequent headache by dilatation of the arteries in the scalp.' This is the claim of vascular theory, but this theory does not explain many aspects of migraine. Another theory states abnormal platelets (clotting particles in blood) cause attacks of migraine. The neural theory says that migraine is due to the primary dysfunction of the brain tissue itself. When a certain threshold is exceeded an attack follows due to a temporary nervous-tissue abnormality. Again there are many shortcomings in this theory, but various brain blood flow studies have shown that there are blood flow changes in brain during a migraine attack. Inflammation cannot be ruled out either. 'Primary nervous system order and a secondary vascular change leading to headaches' is probably what the experts agree as the mechanism of migraine.

Migraine can be triggered by head injuries as in Footballers' Migraine (triggered by heading the ball). Links between epilepsy and migraine have also been noted. Allergic conditions such as asthma, eczema and hay fever have also been linked to migraine but there is no evidence that this is the cause. Nor is there any evidence that migraine is an allergic condition in the accepted medical use of the term. There has been no evidence of 'antibodies' in migraine; and this needs a lot of research work if allergic bases have to be established for migraine.

Treatment of Migraine

1. *Self Help*

The key word to self help for any migraine sufferer is 'understanding'—understanding the condition, the symptoms, etc. Next is analysing factoring causing the attack. The entire family has to cooperate with the patient. If it is not possible to avoid work and lie down at home he can resort to migraine clinics. They offer intra muscular injections of pain killers and drugs to control nausea. At home a dark, quiet place for rest and sleep is required. Thick curtains, eye pads, ear plugs can be helpful. Ice packs or in contrast hot water bottles, both are used to relieve pain.

Migraine can be prevented by avoiding trigger factors. Avoiding the common triggers like chocolate, cheese, citrus fruits or substituting the trigger food (carob for chocolates) can be resorted to by using medical diets (elimination diet). Excessive light is an important trigger factor and can be minimised with sunglasses, visual display units, etc. Modifications in the atmosphere, exercise regime, travel, etc., can all aid in preventing an attack. Stress and anxiety must be decreased; relaxation is important.

Identification of the 'pattern' is very important in the migraine attack management. Predisposing factors like the ones which can be modified should be done. Trigger factors have to be evaluated. Whether they are the avoidable ones, partly avoidable or the unavoidable ones is the main concept to be evaluated.

a) Avoidable trigger factors—sleep, food, pills, H.R. treatment.

b) Partly avoidable triggers—stress, worries, etc.

c) Menstruation.

Certain points have to be paid attention to by the patient. They are (1) nothing can be done about genetic predisposition to migraine. (2) Trigger factors are often multiple. (3) Migraine attacks usually start in the morning and people wake up with it. The reason is not known for this cause. (4) Seasonal variations are seen in migraine. (5) Attacks can occur in cycles, and reason is not known.

Non-drug treatment for migraine includes (1) Meditation, (2) Relaxation programmes like yoga, progressive neuromuscular relaxation, (3) Exercise, (4) Acupuncture, (5) Transcutaneous electrical nerve stimulation (TENS), (6) Aromatherapy, (7) Herbalism, (8) Homoeopathy, (9) Hypnotherapy, (10) Reflexology, (11) Manipulation—osteopathy and chiropractic.

These forms of alternative medicine all differ in their concepts and theories of disease and its treatment. Alternative medicine is a widely used form of therapy for migraine. It is sometimes called Complimentary Medicine to emphasize that it can be used alongwith orthodox medicine—it is not necessarily competing with it.

There are two ways of using drugs to treat migraine—treating the attack once it has started and preventing the attack. The type of drugs used in each case are different.

Pain killers often with a drug to treat sickness are tried first, and only if they are ineffective ergotamine is considered. Soluble preparations work quicker and should be taken early in the attack if there is a warning before the headache. For frequent attacks (two or more a month) it is worth considering daily treatment with preventive drugs. These are not pain killers, they block the effort of various substances on blood vessels or have a direct effect on vessel themselves. They should be tried for several weeks before deciding whether or not they are effective as these drugs work immediately. The most widely used are: Propanolol (Inderal), Pizotitifen (Sanomigran), Clonidine (Dixarit), and Methylsergide (Deseril). They are usually taken for a few months at a time and then discontinued.

Fever few

A popular herb may reduce the frequency and severity of migraines. It contains a compound (parthenolide) that blocks serotonin, a chemical produced by the brain that in excessive amounts may help trigger migraines.

Dose—Chew 2 or 3 leaves or take a standardised extract that has 250 m gms of parthenolide each day to prevent migraines (capsules and tablets may contain little of the active ingredient). Consult your doctor before using fever few to manage migraines. Oral use may cause mouth ulcers and abdominal pain. Not recommended for pregnant women or young children.

Research and Treatment for Migraine

a) These areas of the brain thought to be importance in triggering migraine have been inaccessible so far but recent advances in scanning techniques have given some ideas about this aspect.

b) Migraine is not a disease in the usual meaning of the word. It is a reaction which occurs in predisposed people under certain circumstances. It may be a 'defence reaction' and there is an opinion that it is a way of getting rid of inner tensions but this not been accepted in research circles.

c) Allergic basis of migraine is food acting as a trigger factor for migraine, often generating curiosity regarding whether it has a allergic basis like food allergy, but antibodies are not found for the trigger food. Only future research will give an answer to the allergic basis of the migraine (if any).

d) It is not known what tissue in the body sets off migraine pathways—'brain and neural theory' are being favoured.

e) Chemical study of migraine has shown that many biochemical changes occur in the body and blood vessels. Involvement of prostaglandins, kinins, VA amines, endorphins is suspected. Chemicals like tyramine (a natural substance found in many foods) and flavinoids (present in red wine) are supposed to trigger a migraine attack. This is the suspected chemical in foods causing migraine.

In conclusion we can just say that migraine is a clinical expression in a predisposed person and not a disease and there is no cure for it. As far as its allergic basis is concerned, nothing can be said with conviction until the future research gives conclusive answers.

Summary

1) *Food Allergies :* Allergies have been seen for many food

substances like milk, eggs, nuts, food additives, nuts, fish, etc.

2) *Drug Reactions :* Drugs can produce simple allergic rashes or produce severe anaphylaxis like the penicillin.

3) *Migraine :* Its allergic basis is a highly debated issue. It is precipitated by factors such as food, strong smells, bright light, etc. Neural and vascular mechanisms are being considered as the cause for migraine.

14

TYPES OF HYPERSENSITIVITY REACTIONS

Immunity is the resistance exhibited by the host towards injury caused by micro-organisms and their products. Protection against infectious diseases is only one of the consequences of the immune response which in its entirety is concerned with the reaction of the body against any foreign antigen.

This immunity against infectious diseases can be (1) Innate (2) Acquired. Acquired immunity can be active or passive. They are further classified into cell mediated and humoral, i.e., cells and antibody mediated immunities.

There is considerable confusion in use of the term 'Allergy'. As originally used by Pirquet, allergy meant an altered state of reactivity to an antigen and included both immune responses, namely, protective and injurious. It is still used in this broad sense by some. Others use the term allergy to mean all immune processes harmful to the host, such as hypersensitivity and auto immunity. Allergy is probably most commonly used as a synonym for hypersensitivity. It is sometimes employed in a narrow sense to refer to only one type of hypersensitivity, namely, 'Atopy'.

For induction of the hypersensitivity (allergy) reactions, we have already studied that the host should have contact with an antigen. This will sensitise the immune system leading to formation of antibodies. This is called Priming or Sensitising Dose. Subsequent contact with allergen causes manifestations of hypersensitivity. This is called Shocking Dose host to develop clinical reactions upon re-exposure to antigen. Here we must know what Type I, Type II, Type III and Type IV hypersensitivity reactions are.

Type I	Reaginic	Includes anaphylaxis, atopy
Type II	Cytotoxic	Antibody mediated damages like haemolytic anemia, etc.
Type III	Immune Complex	Arthus reaction, serum sickness
Type IV	Delayed Hypersensitivity	Tuberculin, contact dermatitis

Let us first consider hypersensitivity.

Emergency Kit Items

1) Adrenaline — 1 ml ampoules of 1:1000—five
30ml vial of 1:1000

2) Aminophylline — Ampoules of Aminophylline of 250 mg each

3) Deriphylline — 1 ml ampoules for 1/m injection (5)

4) Anti-histamines — One 10 ml vial of injectable Avil (50 mg/m1)
Avil tablets 25 mg each (10 tabs).

5) Steroids — Decadron 2ml vial (5 vials)
Betnalalan tabs (50 tabs)
Prednisalone tabs (50)

6) Syringes — Tuberulin syringes (2)
2 ml all glass syringes (2 with needles)

7) Tourniquet

The Emergency Kit given above is for anaphylaxis which can

occur due to penicillin injection. Those who are allergic to penicillin are usually also allergic to related drugs like ampicillin and amoxycillin. This must be always kept in mind.

Type I : Reaginic

1. *Anaphylaxis* : We have already learned about it in penicillin-induced allergy. This is a classical immediate hypersensitivity. The term (Ana—without, phylaxis—protection) Anaphylaxis was coined by Ricaet (1902) to describe his observations. As we know, sensitisation is most effective when the antigen is given by injection. The clinical effects of anaphylaxis are due to smooth muscle contraction and increased vascular permeability. Tissues or organs predominantly involved in anaphylactic reaction are known as 'Target Organs'. Other changes seen in Anaphylaxis are oedema, decreased coagulability of blood, fall in BP, fall in temperature, decreased leukocytes and decreased platelets. Cutaneous Anaphlyaxis is when a small shocking dose of an antigen is given intradermally to a sensitised host. There will be a local 'flare and wheal' response (local anaphylaxis). Wheal is a pale central area of puffiness due to oedema, surrounded by flare due to erythema and hypermia. IgE antibodies are the major antibodies involved in hypersensitivity reaction of anaphylaxis. Histamine, serotonin chemotactic factors are the primary mediators of anaphylaxis. PAF, SRS-A, Prostoglandins, leukortriens are all secondary mediators of anaphylaxis.

Intravenous injection of peptone, trypsin, certain other substances provokes a clinical reaction generally resembling anaphylactic shock. This is called Anaphylactoid Reaction. This is a non-specific mechanism, has no immunological basis.

2) *Atopy* : Literally meaning out of place or strangeness it refers to naturally occurring familial hypersensitivities of man typified by hay fever and asthma. Atopy is usually caused by inhalant (pollen dust) or ingestant (food) antigens. IgE antibodies are involved.

Type II : Cytotoxic

These reactions involve the combination of IgE and IgM antibodies. Antigens are on the surface of the cells. The resulting effect is a cytotoxi or cytolytic (cell toxic or cell breaking). Examples are lysis of red cells caused by anti-erythrocyte antibodies in auto immune anemias. Sometimes antigens (drugs) get absorbed to cells. Then the antibodies are formed for this and a reaction ensues. Drug induced purpura (bleeding) falls under this type II reactions. Antigens can be either the cell itself or a substance absorbed into the cells. The first category has given rise to the concept of 'Auto Immunity', literally meaning 'protection against self' while it actually implies 'Injury to self' because in this condition structural or functional damage is produced by the action of immunologically competent cells or antibodies against normal components of the body. Therefore, the term Auto Immunity has been criticised as contradiction in terms. 'Auto allergy' has been suggested as an acceptable alternative but the term 'Auto Immunity' has the sanction of wide usage. When the concept of auto immunity came to be accepted as a pathogenic mechanism a large number of diseases were suggested to have an auto immune actiology based on the finding of auto (self) antibodies in the patients. This was recognised to be untenable as auto antibodies could be often the result and not the cause of the disease. Therefore, there are certain guidelines for a disease to be declared as auto immune. They are (1) the auto immune response must be regularly associated with the disease. (2) the antigen responsible must be identified, insolated and characterised. (3) the same antigen must induce in experimental animals the immune pathological changes of disease it has been implicated to cause. (4) passive transfer of the disease must be possible by the transfer of antibodies.

Auto Immune (Auto allergic) diseases usually show (1) demonstrable antibodies, (2) an elevated levels of various immunoglobulins, and (3) the person having the disease has usually more than one auto immune pathology.

1) Hidden antigens may get recognised as self-antigens

2) Cells or tissues undergo antigenic alterations due to physical, chemical, biological agents forming 'Neo-antigens'

Immune cells, antibody defects also contribute to autoimmunity

They enter circulation and indue an immune response

Results in production against body's own hidden/neo-antigens

"Auto Immunity" damages body's own tissues/organs

He shows improvement with steroid and immunosuppressive treatment and a genetic predisposition towards auto immunity.

Mechanism of Auto Immunity or Auto Allergy : There are many many auto immune diseases :

a) *Auto Immune Haemolytic Anemias* : Auto antibodies against RBCs of Blood are found in patient. This destroys RBCs prematurely in spleen and liver leading to anemia.

b) *Auto Immune Thrombocytopenia* : Here antibodies are seen for platelets (also called thrombocytes) which leads to destruction of platelets and consequent haemorrhage in the form of purpura.

c) *Auto Immune Leucopenia* : Antibodies against WBCS (leukocytes) seen in rheumatoid arthritis.

d) *Auto Immune Thyrotoxicosis (Graves Disease) and Hashimotos Disease* : Auto immune diseases affecting the thyroid gland.

Antibodies for thyroglobulin is seen in both cases. Graves disease and hashimotos (this is a form of Goitre; enlarged thyroid gland) have been studied extensively. Hashimotos affects females more and is characterised by symptoms of hypo (low) thyroidism, i.e., decreased activity of the thyroid gland.

e) *Addison's Disease* : Antibodies against the cells of adrenal gland are seen.

f) *Auto Immune Orchitis* : Antibodies to sperms, germinal cells leading to aspermatogenesis (no production of sperm).

g) *Myasthenia Gravis* : Abnormal fatigue of muscles. Antibodies to muscles are seen in serum (anti-muscle antibodies). [Film actor Amitabh Bachchan suffered from this pathology.]

h) *Pernicious Anemia* : Antibodies are present against gastric mucosa cells leading to anemia by complex mechanisms.

i) *Auto Immune Diseases of Eye* : Antibodies to lens during cataract surgery can occur leading to ocular inflammation-called Phacoanaphylaxis. Auto Immune diseases of the nervous system like Idiophatic (cause unknown) *Polyneuritis* is considered to be auto immune in nature in which antibodies to the peripheral nervous tissue are implicated. Following rabies vaccination there can be neuroparalytic reactions. This is due to antibodies against sheep nervous tissue. A general experimental allergic encephalmyelitis can be produced in animals with the nervous tissue extract.

j) *Systemic Auto Immune Diseases* : This includes conditions characterised by a variety of self-antigens inducing formation of antibodies leading to immune response and resulting in damage to several organs and tissue systems. This group includes :

i) Systemic Lupus Erythematosus (SLE)

ii) Rheumatoid Arthritis (RA)

iii) Polyarteritis Nodosa (PN)

iv) Sjogren's Syndrome (SS)

i) In the SLE, auto immune has been studied with great interest. This is a chronic, multisystem disease with remissions and exacerbations terminating fatally. Auto antibodies are found against cell nuclei, intracrytoplasmic cell constituents, immunoglobulins, thyroid and many other components. Certain antibodies have been found which are directed against organ specific antigens. There are the very characteristic anti-DNA (antinuclear) antibodies. The 'Lupus Erythematosus' phenomenon (LE phenomenon) are the cells with typical constituents. A complete breakdown of the 'Immunological' balance is suggested in SLE. Clinical symptoms include rashes, oral ulcers, photo sensitivity, renal, hemalologic, immunologic neurologic disorders, arthritis, pleurits, pericarditis, etc.

ii) RA, Symmetric Poly (many) Arthritis (inflammation of joints), muscle wasting, subcutaneous nodules, associated with myocarditis, etc., are common in adult females. Auto antibodies called 'Rheumatoid Factors' (RF) are seen against a particular part of Immunoglobulin IgG. The "IgG-RF" in particular is of interest because it is a rare instance in which the same molecule functions as the 'Antigen and Antibody'.

iii) PN (Polyartiritis Nodesa) is a disease of medium-sized arteries. There is inflammation and destruction (Necrotising angitis). This leads to a block in coronary arteries, cerebral haemorrhage, gIt bleeding, etc. Auto antibodies are yet to be detected.

iv) In Sjogren's Syndrome the symptoms can be conjuctivitis and dryness, dry mouth, rheumatoid arthiritis plus there may be salivary gland enlargement. Antibodies against nucleus of cells and RF are seen in serum.

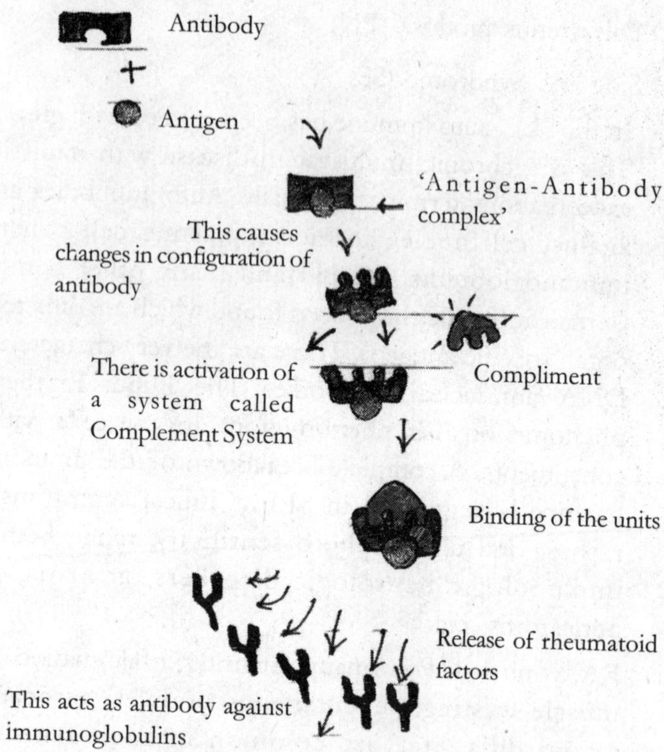

Fig. 14.1 : Auto Immune Basic Increase Mechanism Involved in R. Arthritis

Apart from the various auto immune diseases mentioned above, there can be certain conditions like drug therapy, infections, etc., which can bring transitory auto immune responses.

3) *Type III Immune Complex Diseases*

This is the third category in the classification of allergic or hypersensitivity reactions. This includes :

i) *Arthus Reaction* : Arthus (1903) observed that when rabbits were injected with normal horse serum repeatedly, subcutaneously the initial injections were without any local effect, but with later injections, there occurred intense local reaction consisting of oedema (fluid retention), induration and haemorrhagic necrosis (destruction). This is called Arthus Reaction and is due to the formation of the 'Antigen-Antibody' precipitates which deposit on the blood vessel walls.

ii) *Serum Sickness* : As originally described by Von Pirquet and Schick (1905) this appeared 7-12 days following a single injection of high concentration of foreign serum such as diphtheria antiserum. The clinical syndrome consists of fever, spleen and lympho node enlargements, inflammation of kidney (nephritis), blood-vessels, joints (arthritis), urticarial rashes, nausea, vomiting, and abdominal pain. The pathogensis is formation of immune complexes (consisting of foreign serum and antibody to it that reaches high enough titres by 7-12 days). These get deposited on blood vessel walls in various parts of body, producing inflammation. The disease is self-limited with subsequent injections. The disease manifests earlier.

Serum sickness differs from other types of hypersensitivity reactions in that a single injection can serve as both a Sensitising and Shocking dose. As heterologous serum injections are not used often now, the syndrome in more commonly seen following injections of penicillin or other antibiotics. Immune complexes (i.e., antigen-antibody complexes) occur in many diseases including bacterial, viral, parasitic infections, etc.

Type IV Delayed Hypersensitivity

They are provoked by specific antigens, evolve slowly and involve immune cells like lymphocytes and macrophages. The reaction is not by circulating antibodies, but by sensitised T cells which react with antigen, release chemicals called Lymphokines (these produce biological effects on the W.B.C.S.) and bring about the delayed hypersensitivity.

The other type of delayed hypersensitivity is Tuberculin (or infection) Type. When a small dose of tuberculin is injected intradermally in an individual sensitised to tuberculo protein prior infection or immunisation an indurated inflammatory reaction occurs at site within 48-72 hours. In unsensitised individuals, there is no response to tuberculin infection. This test provides useful indication of the state of delayed HS to the bacippus (Tuberculous bacillus is the bacterial causing TB. 'Tuberculin is the protein of TB bacillus). Tuberculin type of HS is seen in infections with bacteria, virus, fungi, parasites. A similar hypersensitivity also develops in allograft reaction.

What is a shwartyman reaction? Shwartyman observed that if a culture filtrate of salmonella typhi bacteria was infected intradermally in a rabbit, after 24 hours again the filtrate was given by IV, there was a haemorrhagic necrotic lesion on the intradermal site. This kind of reactions (called shwartyman reaction) has no immunological basis. It is due to the alteration in factors affecting the intravascular coagulation. They are described with hypersensitivity states because they resemble them superficially and one should be able to distinguish *it* from hypersensitive states.

Summary

1) Immediate and delayed are the basic classes of allergic reactions. Type 1, Type II, Type III, Type IV are the four types of hypersensitivity reactions.

2) Arthus reaction, serum sickness, tuberculin reactions are all discussed.

3) Reactions to pure proteins and haemorhagic allergic states have been briefly discussed.

4) Antigen-Antibody reaction, the very basis of allergy, and all the immune reactions have been discussed in connection with transplantation, transfusion, malignancies.

5) Auto Immune or Auto Allergy conditions are very important as these are conditions in which antibodies are produced against the own antigens (normal components of body) causing damage to structure/function.

15

IMMUNOTHERAPY AND ALLERGIC CONJUNCTIVITIS

Allergic conjunctivitis has always been mentioned along with allergic rhinitis. The logic behind including the Allergic conjunctivitis alongwith Immunotherapy is that:

1) Immunotherapy is being used more and more in the treatment of allergic conjunctivitis.
2) Both immunotherapy and allergic conjunctivitis are 'hot' and 'happening' topics in allergic seminars.

Immunity from Allergies : Revolutionary Treatment

Experts from all over the world gathered in Kuala Lumpur recently for the fifth Malaysian Conference of Allergy and Immunology. One of the important topics discussed in this conference was immunotherapy. For those who have to buy special mattress covers, clean their house religiously and get rid of their pets just to stay allergy free, an "allergy vaccine" would most certainly be a Godsend.

Allergy vaccination, also known as Immunotherapy, has revolutionised the treatment of allergy. Traditionally allergy treatment only controlled the symptoms of allergy, but could not reverse or prevent the disease. Currently available medication for allergic diseases is effective in improving symptoms, but does not change the natural history of the diseases. The goal of immunotherapy is to induce long-term tolerance to allergens.

Immunotherapy is being developed as a long-term effective treatment for allergic disorders. A statistics predicts that by the time Malaysia would achieve the developed status in 2020 almost half of its population would have developed some form of allergy.

We all know that allergy is a hyper-reactivity to normal harmless environmental substances. When these allergens enter the body of an allergic person, his immune system overreacts and produces antibodies to fight these antigens. These antibodies attack allergy cells which produce histamines and produce symptoms of allergy.

Immunotherapy modifies the body's allergic response by gradually exposing one to high levels of a particular allergen and helping his body to build a tolerance to it. Eventually his immune reaction towards that allergen is reduced. This novel form of treatment uses purified allergens in liquid form that are introduced into the body through a series of subcutaneous injections or sublingual mouth drops.

Imagine five vials filled with liquid (say, dustmite). Each vial is marked with a number 0, 1, 2, 3, 4. The number 0 is the smallest dose and 4 is the highest dose.

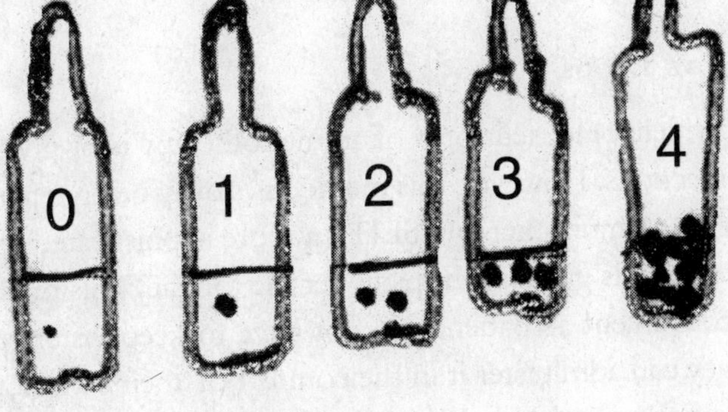

Fig. 15.1 : Vials having allergen in increasing levels of potency

The current immunotherapy can only treat allergic rhinitis (allergy in nose) and allergic conjunctivitis (allergy in the eyes) and allergic asthma arising from aero allergens like house dust, mites, cat and dog dander, pollen. Immunotherapy can also protect against bee and wasp venom anaphylaxis, but not against skin and food allergies. Many doctors feel that life certainly becomes better for their patients on immunotherapy. Allergic symptoms and drug consumption both go down. The quality of the patients' life improved and their general resistance increased. At the end of the course, patients we either able to go off their medication completely or reduce it substantially. The patient is expected to be immune to that allergen for eight to 10 years. The earlier one starts the immunotherapy the better. Children respond very quickly. A two year-old will lose the allergy within four months while an adult will need six to eight months. But very little is known about the immune response after the 10-years mark but certain points are assured :

1) a general decrease in overall allergies
2) a decrease in development of new allergies
3) a decrease in other allergies that the person might have even though he was not treated for it.

Injections vs Drops

The most widely practised form of immunotherapy is by giving a series of injections. However, this method is slowly being replaced by Sublingual Immunotherapy (SLIT), a more sophisticated form of treatment that is given as drops under the tongue. This method is highly convenient as patients do not have to keep visiting the doctor. They can administer it in the comfort of their own home. It is also painless and kids love it because it tastes nice. While

SLIT and injections are both effective, the latter has the added risk that a severe reaction may occur during the injection. Several deaths have occurred from the use of injections due to untrained personnel giving the treatment, without having the proper facilities to deal with emergencies. Injectable immunotherapy has to be given by a fully trained physician within a setting of good resuscitation facilities. Injections are still necessary for insect venom immunotherapy.

SLIT is an extremely safe and effective method of immunotherapy causing only minor side effects. It causes itching of the tongue, lips and mouth but it only lasts for a few seconds. There is also the occasional tummy ache, which is very rare. This can be prevented if you take drops at the same time every day, half an hour before a meal.

Receiving the Treatment

The current trend is that very strict selection criteria were used in prescribing immunotherapy. The patient has to have a confirmed moderate to severe allergy. It is not suitable for people with mild allergies, like those who have the odd itchy nose or sniff once a month. The main thing is accurate identification of what the person is allergic to. The doctor must also make sure that there is nothing else that can be contributing to that allergy. Blood tests are a way to identify allergies as they measure the amount of IgE antibodies in the blood and give an indication of how severe the allergy is. When a patient has been identified as suitable for immunotherapy, he will take daily drops at gradually increasing doses. After that he moves on to the maintenance phase, where he continues taking the highest dose of the vaccine thrice a week for up to three years. Throughout the three years, the patients are monitored to make sure they do not have any serious side effects. The patients have to stay on their prescribed allergy treatment (such as antihistamines and steroids) as well as continue avoiding allergens until they become hyposensitised.

Naturally, there are those who stop the treatment when they start feeling better. Some patients start feeling much better after a few months or one year. So getting them to finish the next two years is a bit of a problem. Although the patient feels better it is only temporary. He has to complete the three years or the allergy will come straight back. He has to be serious when he embarks on immunotherapy. It cannot be treated as a joke.

Immunotherapy is expensive. Sublingual immunotherapy (SLIT) is cost effective, and in the long run reduces the need for rhinitis and asthma medication. Government hospitals must take up immunotherapy as patients visit such hospitals more than private clinics.

Allergic Conjunctivitis

There is a light breeze outside and you open the windows to enjoy the fresh air. Suddenly your child's eyes start streaming and he rubs them with his knuckles. 'Mom, it's itchy,' he complains, still rubbing away madly. You brush his hands away to take a look at his eyes. To your horror, not only are they red and watery they are almost swollen shut. Tiny, near invisible pollen blown in from the garden had 'attacked' your child, causing an allergic reaction in his eyes known as Allergic Conjunctivitis.

Allergic conjunctivitis is a broad group of allergic conditions involving inflammation of the conjunctiva. The conjunctiva is the thin membrane that covers the surface of the inner eyelid and part of the eyeball. The surface of the eye is the most obviously exposed mucous membrane of the body. Unlike the nose and lungs, the eyes have no filtration devices (like cilia, the tiny hairs on the surface of a cell) for expelling allergens. The defence mechanism in the eye is the tear film which provides a barrier, and dilutes and rinses away allergens. Most cells, those responsible for causing an allergic response, are concentrated in certain parts of the body like the nose, lungs, skin, eyes and digestive system. If a person is prone to allergies, he is more likely to get a reaction in one or more of these organs. If the inflammation (or reaction) occurs in the nose, it is called Rhinitis; in the lungs, it is called Asthma and in the eyes, it is called Conjunctivitis. The typical symptoms of allergic conjunctivitis are pronounced itching, redness, watery or ropy discharge. However, people often dismiss these symptoms and instead pay more attention to treating their rhinitis (known as hay fever, if seasonal). This is why allergic conjunctivitis is sometimes left untreated leading to complications that threaten the eyesight.

Of all the different parts of one's eyes, the cornea is the one which is to be worried about. Two types of allergic conjunctivitis—Vernal or Atopic Kerato Conjunctivitis—may affect the cornea. If the cornea becomes damaged, it can affect one's sight. Other complications that could develop are glaucoma or even loss of vision which occur if the use of steroids is not carefully monitored.

The most common form of eye allergies is intermittent or seasonal allergic conjunctivitis (see the Table for different types of allergic conjunctivitis). Seasonal allergic conjunctivitis affects 5 to 22 per cent of the general population. It often co-exists with hay fever, up to one-third or half of the patients with hay fever may also have conjunctivitis. Allergic conjunctivitis typically sets in at an early age with more than 80 per cent of patients affected before the age of 30.

Table 15.1 : Types of Allergic Conjunctivitis

Type	*Description*	*Causes*	*Symptoms*
1) Acute allergic conjunctivitis	Sudden onset of allergic reaction that occurs at any age, especially childhood	When large quantities of an allergen, such as pollen, enter the eye	Intense itching
2) Intermitten or seasonal allergic conjunctivitis	A seasonal allergy that is frequently associated with allergic rhinitis (rhino conjuntivitis)	Seasonal allergens, typically pollen	Itching of the eyes, watering and redness; signs of hyperaemia (excess of blood) and oedema (accumulation of fluid) in lower eyelid.
3) Persistent/ perennial conjunctivitis	A mild chronic form of allergic conjunctivitis	Continual exposure to perennial allergen such as house dust, mites, moulds, animal and cockroach allergens	Itching, watering and redness
4) Giant conjunctivitis	A condition caused by mechanical trauma, does not involve the cornea	Trauma caused by contact lenses, ocular prosthese or post-operative sutures; may be aggravated by concomitant allergy	Giant (bigger than 1mm in diameter; papillary growth on the upper eyelid

(Contd. ...)

Type	Description	Causes	Symptoms
5) Vernal conjunct-ivitis	A severe inflam-matory disease, may be seasonal or persistent; usually occurs in childhood and early adolescence; more in males than in females	May be caused by genetic factors upon awaking; pain; blurred vision and sens-	Watering and itching of eyes; stickiness; difficulty in opening eyelids itivity to light (if cornea is involved)
6) Atopic kerato conjunct-ivitis	A severe lifelong disease starting in young adult-hood, more fre-quently in males. If it is neglected the cornea can be sight-threatening	Associated with atopic eczema/ dermatitis syn-drome; infarction, corneal thinning; cataracts; eye in-fection; may be exacerbated by contact with allergens.	Persistent itching of eyes; eye soreness; impaired vision; dryness of eye; copious mucous dis-charge; eyelids may be glued shut upon awaking.

Source : *Allergic Conjunctivitis Revised Guidelines*, June 2003, GLORIA-WAO.

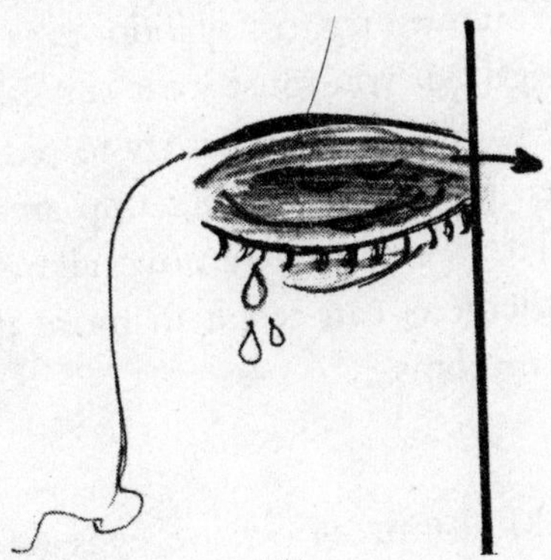

Fig. 15.2 : Oedema in Conjunctivitis

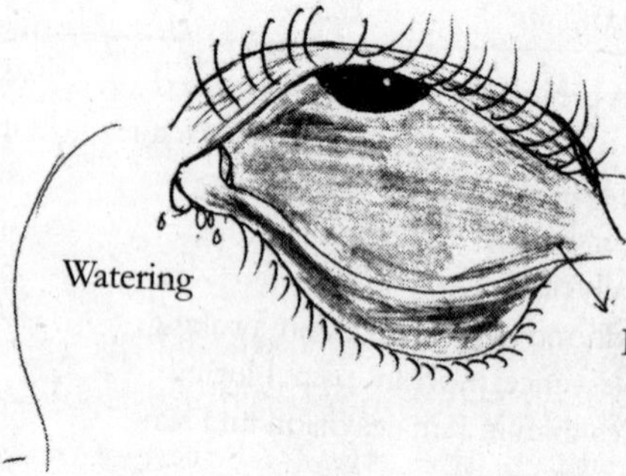

Fig. 15.3 : Allergic Conjunctivitis

Preventing an Attack

The first step in managing allergic conjunctivitis and any other form of allergy is allergen avoidance and environmental control. House dust, mites, grass, tree and weed pollen, pet dander, cockroaches and moulds are frequently involved in allergic conjunctivitis. Tobacco smoke, indoor gases, and environmental pollutants from automobiles can aggravate allergic symptoms.

Maintain hygiene in the home. Change and wash your bedding regularly. Remove or reduce contact with pets and stuffed toys and get rid of cockroaches in the house. It is difficult to avoid pollen altogether. You must try to stay indoors as much as possible and if you have to go out you must wear sunglasses and a hat. If a person is allergic to mould, he must try to reduce the humidity in the house so that there will be less damp areas. It may not be possible to completely avoid or remove allergens. But even a reduction in the allergens can result in more than 30 per cent improvement in symptoms.

Treating Itchy Eyes

One can use a cold compress on the eyes to soothe mild to moderate symptoms like itching and swelling. Preservative free tear drops (artificial tears) are another effective and inexpensive form of over-the-counter therapy. The teardrops moisten the eye and ease irritation. They prove to be even more soothing if they are refrigerated. If these do not work one may have to resort to medications, like the following:

1) Topical non-steroidal anti-inflammatory drugs (in the form of eyedrops). One type is ketoropac promethamine used to relieve itching, redness, oedema, photophobia, foreign body sensation, and discharge. However, the effect of illness of ketorolac is limited.

2) Vaso-constrictors which cause narrowing of blood vessels can be applied to reduce redness in the eyes. These are not recommended for daily use.

3) Topical anti-histamines can be used to relieve itching and redness. This is a safe and effective form of therapy for children three years and older. When combined with vaso-constrictor, these agents are fast acting but do not provide day-long relief. Oral anti-histamines are a popular form of medication for other allergies like rhinitis but they may not be as useful in allergic conjunctivitis. They are less effective than topical anti-histamines and may cause the unwanted 'dry eye' effect, exacerbating the irritation in the eyes. Unlike the other medications that treat the symptoms, topical mast cell stabilisers prevent an allergic reaction by preventing the release of histamine and other meditators from mast cells. Most mast cell stabilisers work effectively but they do not act immediately; neither do they work if an allergic reaction has already begun.

Newer allergy drugs combine the action of anti-histamines and mast cell stabilisers (also known as dual-action antihistamine/ mast cell stabilisers).

These are more effective in relieving symptoms than medication alone and can also be used to prevent the onset of symptoms. One form of treatment that requires careful use is topical corticosteroids. Steroids should be used only in cases of severe (not intermittent or seasonal) allergic conjunctivitis. They must be prescribed and monitored by an ophthalmologist. Prolonged use can lead to secondary bacterial infection, glaucoma, cataracts, and delayed wound healing.

The other potentially harmful effects of steroids is that it may be prescribed in the wrong situation, for instance, for a patient who has an eye infection instead of an allergy. The use of steroids may aggravate the problem, even leading to loss of vision.

A relatively new form of allergy treatment is immuno-therapy which can be used to manage perennial allergic conjunctivitis and atopic kerato conjunctivitis. Eye allergies are not something one should brush aside. At best it will cause a great deal of misery. At worst it may lead to serious eye complications that could cost a person his vision. If a doctor has a patient with allergic rhinitis, he must think beyond the nose.

Summary

1. Immunotherapy has become very sophisticated and is the line of treatment for certain forms of allergies.
2. SLIT (Sublingual Immunotherapy) has its own merits and advantages.
3. Allergic conjunctivitis should get individual attention. It is not to be always treated with or discussed with allergic rhinitis. It has its own identity and needs treatment of symptoms and causes as a separate entity.
4. Immunotherapy is the treatment in certain forms of allergic conjunctivitis.
5. Allergic conjunctivitis and immunotherapy have become important, current happening 'topics' of discussion in allergy conferences and symposiums.

16

NEW TRENDS IN ALLERGY TREATMENT

Wheeze Relief

There is a new non-steroidal treatment for childhood asthma with few side effects. The pain of a child who is suffering from an asthma attack is very stressful. Indeed one would have to be stone-hearted not to be moved by the sight of a child coughing and wheezing, and having difficulty in breathing. But if it is any consolation to parents, doctors say it is very rare for death to occur in an asthma attack and many children with asthma at a young age may outgrow it, although some symptoms may reappear later in life. The trauma of childhood asthma is often a topic of great importance discussed in various medical seminars and symposiums. There is a non-new steroidal oral medication for asthmatic children between the ages of two and five. Medically termed 'Montelukast Sodium' the new once-a-day tablet provides effective asthma control to asthmatic children in that age group, according to recent global study.

Traditionally worldwide, only bronchodilators are used which act by relaxing and dilating the air passages. Inhalation is the common way to administer them but the problem with bronchodilators is that they sometimes relieve the symptoms, but do not treat the disease.

We all know that three things happen in an asthma attack: the muscles around the tubes that carry air to the lungs contract and narrow the airways; then the glands produce more mucus; and the lining of the tubes are inflamed. If the inflammation is not treated then the disease is not treated. Montelukast has been found to treat all the three conditions.

It is difficult for asthmatic children under five years of age to learn how to use an inhaler. The convenience and tolerability of the new tablet is a boon to them. This tablet is chewable and cherry coloured. A study was conducted in 93 hospitals all over the world. In the study of 689 asthmatic children aged two to five it was found the montelukast significantly reduced a broad range of symptoms and reduced parameters of asthmatic inflammation. The drug also improved daytime asthma symptoms which included severity of coughs, wheezing, trouble in breathing and activity limitations. The study also evaluated the safety and tolerability of montelukast (4 mg) and placebo administered once daily at bedtime in the 689 boys and girls with physician-diagnosed asthma. It was a randomised control trial where 200 children took the placebo and 400 children took the drug. A daily card was given to facilitators to fill in the daily symptoms of each child for three months. The results showed that children receiving montelukast had less coughing, less wheezing and were more active. They also had few attacks of breathlessness. The drug is not very fast, less faster than bronchodilators but it can be used with the existing treatment and it treats inflammation.

Prof. Dr. John Price, the clinical Director of Paediatrics at Kings College Hospital in London, has talked extensively on childhood asthma and montelukast's efficiency. He says that prevalence in childhood asthma varies in different countries. The highest number of cases is in the UK, Australia, NewZealand, while the lowest is in India and Eastern Europe.

In Malaysia studies show that some 30 per cent of asthmatic children will have developed symptoms by two years of age and

80 per cent by the age of five. At least 1.8 million Malaysians suffer from asthma, with children and young adults comprising the most common groups of asthma sufferers. About half of all preschool children (in the entire world) wheeze at some point and four out of 10 will stop wheezing by the time they go to school, says Dr. Price.

As it is not easy to tell whether asthma is transient or chronic, doctors will have to decide whether to give treatment and how often as well as how much to give. Trying to decide whether the asthma will go away or not is not the point. The point is to determine whether a child needs treatment, and once he is started on treatment, is it important to monitor the progress. The aim of the treatment is to make the child sleep through the night without coughing or wheezing. For the children with severe symptoms inhaling steroids is the answer though this does not always work well. In serious cases, it is recommended that montelukast be added to their existing treatment of inhaled steroids as both medicines have been proven to be a good combination. No serious side effects have been reported for this new drug except for the occasional headache.

Generally there are two groups of asthmatic children. One group just wheezes and has colds with no allergies with no other family member suffering the same disease, while the other group comprises children who have persistent asthma and develop allergies. The second group also tends to include family members suffering the same fate. Exact distinction between the two groups is not yet known. It could be genetics or the environment. Apart from the 'treatment at the moment', the single most important thing in preventing severe asthma is to ensure that the child does not breathe in second-hand smoke. Smoking during pregnancy can double the likelihood of wheezing attacks for a child during the first three years of his life.

Though at present there is no cure for asthma, with proper management and treatment children with asthma can lead normal and active lives.

Fish Oil in Preventing Allergies

Fish oil supplements taken during pregnancy might help prevent allergies in babies at high risk for them, a preliminary research suggests. A study in Australia found that babies whose mothers took fish oil had weaker immune reactions to common allergy triggers and at one year of age showed signs of being less allergy prone.

Omega 3 Fatty Acids

Anti-inflammatory properties

Effects on 'immune' system of the body

Makes it less prone to allergic reactions

(*Times of India Report*)

The new study looked at whether Fish Oil Capsules—rich in healthful omega 3 fatty acids—might help prevent allergies in babies born to women, with a history of hay fever or asthma risk, of developing them. The theory is that because omega 3 fatty acids have anti-inflammatory properties, they may affect the developing immune system in a way that makes it less prone to allergic reactions, according to studies conducted by Dr. Susan L. Prescott of the University of Western Australia in Perth. However, she says that this is the first study to look at this in very early life and so more work is clearly needed. These findings have been published in the *Journal of Allergy and Clinical Immunology*. Prescott's team had 98 pregnant women take either fish oil capsules or for comparison capsules containing olive oil. Analysing cells taken from the babies' umbilical cord, blood, greater amounts of omega 3 fats were found in the cell membranes of newborns whose mothers took fish oil supplements.

Nutrients to ward off Allergies

Eating right can help a lot. It is not just about avoiding what is wrong for you. Actually the right food can help you keep your allergies at bay. There are lots of nutrients that can help you. These are stuff that you find in wholesome and fresh foods. Among the most important is an essential fatty acid that basically comes from fish. It is called Omega 3 Fatty Acid. Taking lots of omega 3 fatty acid (Ω3FA) keeps allergy away. Taking high doses of it even helps to suppress the inflammatory response the way steroids do, but without the associated side effects.

The big breakthrough in our understanding of omega 3 and its powerful influences on body physiology came about following Nobel Prize-winning research in 1982. As the omega 3 family of carbon chain molecules is involved in the production of Eicosanoids it can have steroid-like effects without the side effects of steroids. They can help calm inflammation and reduce the immune response of the immune system. In inhibiting the production of "bad" eicosanoids and becoming the raw material for the production of "good" eicosanoids, fish oils exert many beneficial effects. As steroids and aspirins inhibit the process in the eicosanoids production, they inhibit the production of all eicosanoids—both good and bad—leading to serious side effects. In order to suppress the production of 'bad' eicosanoids you need to have high doses. Also these high doses are needed because in a diseased state, the eicosanoid status is badly out of balance. You need to dramatically boost the levels of the 'good' eicosanoids to counter the 'bad' eicosanoids. Powerful anti- inflammatory effects of EPA are best demonstrated in allergic disorders. The overactive immune system can be calmed by doses of EPA and DHA in excess of 3 gm on just a few weeks. This has been demonstrated clinically. This can be invaluable for the patients suffering from allergies.

Sources

Most people think that the omega 3 fatty acids in fish body oil are produced by the fish themselves. They are wrong! The fish do not produce (cannot produce either) any of these long chain fatty acids themselves. Only Micro-algae can produce these long and complex long chain fatty acids. Fish merely consume the fatty acids produced by microalgae that thrive deep in the ocean at the base of the marine foodchain. This is especially so of cold water fish that have lots of body fat to keep them warm and alive in icy waters. Nutritional experts have learned that Omega 3 oils are vitally important during all phases of life. They also believe that a person's diet should include oily fish, several times per week. Omega 2 FA are an excellent alternative for those who do not eat fish frequently or who would like to ensure a high intake of these essential polyunsaturated fatty acids (EPA).

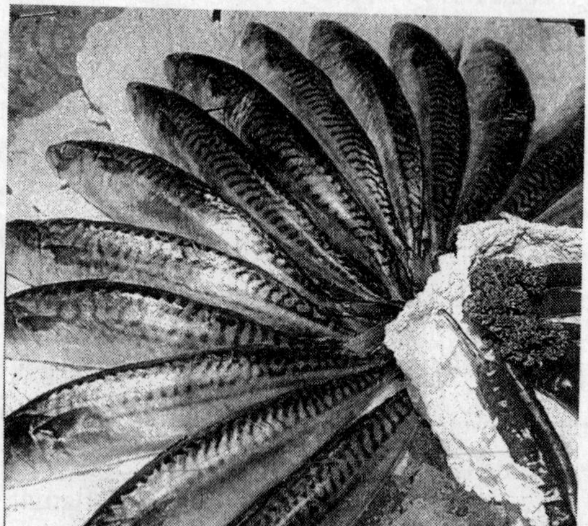

Fig. 16.1 : Oily Fish like the Blue Mackerel

Oily fish like the Blue Mackerel are rich in omega 3 and should be included in the diet several times per week.

Supplements

If you do not take fish regularly, you can supplement with fish oil capsules. Children too need fish oil. However, giving pure fish oil to kids has always been a problem. Despite attempts to mask the taste by using different flavours, parents are still finding it difficult to make their children take fish oil.

Soft gelatine omega 3 capsules are easier to handle. The capsules may be leaked into a chocolate flavoured drink that rather effectively masks the taste and smell. More recently, chewable fish oil tablets that taste of fish, but with minimal smell, have become available in pharmacile.

Toxins

However, taking fish oil supplements can be dangerous in itself. The oceans are increasingly contaminated. In 2001 the State of Massachusetts even advised pregnant women not to eat fish. There has been a lot of concern over mercury contamination and hence pregnant women and children are advised to restrict their fish intake to eight ounces/week. Environmental organisations have conducted analysis of many brands of fish oils in various countries of the world and have found that they contain high levels of toxins—DDT, PCB, lindane, oranochlorine pesticides. Sometimes taking even therapeutic doses of these oils can lead to toxicity due to polluntants. Molecularly distilled fish oils are to be used. This is a high tech process that allows the removal of all toxins without affecting the highly sensitive fish oil. Allergic reactions could result in symptoms involving the nose (rhinitis), skin (atopic dermatitis), eyes (conjunctivitis) or lungs (asthma). Hence it is very vital that proper treatment is instituted. Allergic rhinitis should not be ignored because it can severely disrupt a person's enjoyment of life. In one airway survey conducted for the European Federation of Allergy and Airway Diseases Patients Association, over 80 per cent of Asian parents interviewed said that asthma and allergy manifestations such as allergic rhinitis disrupted their children's daily activities at home and in school.

Prof. Ruby, who is the Chairperson of the ARIA (Allergic Rhinitis and its Impact on Asthma), WHO initiative in the Asia-Pacific, points out that, allergic rhinitis has ever been found to increase the risk of developing asthma. Unfortunately, allergic diseases are not well treated in Asia due to limited awareness of its prevalence and dangers.

Allergic Asia

The allergic manifestations are aggravated by environmental polluntants. There are indoor polluntants, like tobacco smoke, kerosene, smoke from wood fuel and formaldehyde as well as outdoor pollutants like CO and So_2. Certain people have a tendency to become (atopic) allergic. Almost 40 per cent of the world's population is atopic. Asia-Pacific already covers half of the world population, so half of the global burden of allergic diseases lies in Asia. There has been an increase in the prevalence of allergic diseases all over the world even in developing countries. This is explained by the fact that the incidence of allergies rises during the process of development. Most Asian countries are in the process of development. So we see a sudden marked rise. The incidence is very high, on average 10-40 per cent.

Latest researches on allergic rhinitis show that it is the most common form of allergic disease. It is an allergic response in the nose mediated by release of chemicals like leukotrienes, prostaglandins, histamines producing various symptoms. Allergic rhinitis is classified as intermittent or the persistent type. Intermittent rhinitis is nothing but the hay fever which occurs mostly in USA and Europe. Moderate severe persistent rhinitis is the most predominant form of allergy in Asia. The criteria for distinguishing allergic rhinitis from common cold are itchy nose and itchy eyes. If there is fever, it is not an allergy. Allergic rhinitis affects the quality of life and it is also a risk factor for asthma. Allergic rhinitis increases the risk of developing asthma by three times. About 80 per cent of the asthmatic patients have allergic rhinitis. In children, more than 80 per cent of asthmatic children have their condition due to allergies.

Patients with persistent allergic rhinitis should be evaluated for asthma, especially if they have symptoms like an irritating cough or light wheezing. Generally patients with asthma should be evaluated for rhinitis.

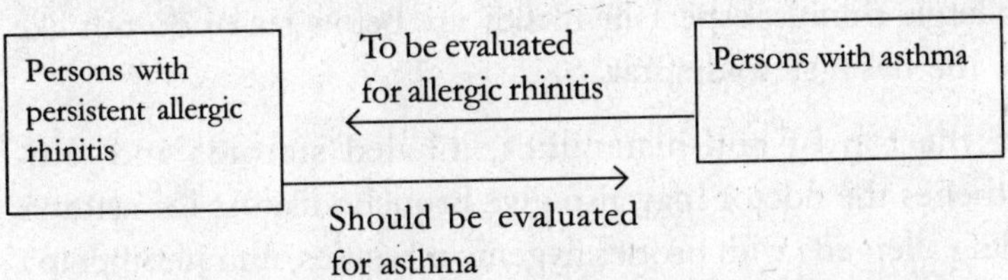

Some people do not see the need to treat allergic rhinitis when it has not led to asthma. But neglecting the symptoms of allergic rhinitis not only worsens the patient's physical condition but also burdens him financially. There is increasing evidence that patients not treated for allergic rhinitis have a 61 per cent increased chance of being hospitalised compared to those who receive treatment. There are many safe and effective drugs that can control allergic rhinitis. However the treatment for allergic rhinitis should take into account the presence of asthma and vice versa. If the doctor only treats the lower airways (asthma) by giving more and more steroids, it does not solve the problem of the upper airways. Hence the concept of "One Airway One Disease". The two conditions are treated together.

Allergic rhinitis can be treated with anti-histamines and steroids. There are first generation and second-generation anti-histamines. Older first generation should be avoided as they cause heavy sedation, and side effects are harmful to patients with asthma. Topical nasal sprays of steroids are the most commonly used. Asthma (if present) needs inhaled steroids to clear lower airways. While nasal steroids and inhaled steroids are safe individually, parents are still worried about the total amount of steroids given to their children.

Anti-leukotrienes, which are non-steroidal oral drugs, can be used as an alternative to the nasal steroids. They have shown to be safe and effective for both allergic rhinitis and asthma. By cutting down on the nasal steroids one is reducing the total load of steroids. Anti-leukotrienes can also be given to patients with only allergic rhinitis, especially if they are below six or do not like to use the nasal steroid spray.

On the top of anti-histamines, inhaled steroids and anti-leukotrienes the doctor may also give bronchodilators for asthma. Avoiding allergens with proper hygenic measures, immunotherapy, surgery also feature in the treatment of allergic rhinitis if needed. Allergic rhinitis is a huge socioeconomic burden. In the USA alone US $ 3 billion has been spent on the treatment of allergic rhinitis. However, not treating is even more expensive. Cost should not be a reason to sacrifice adequate and effective treatment.

Summary

1) There is a new non-steroidal treatment for childhood asthma with few side effects called 'Montelukast'. It is a chewable tablet, hence easy to administer to children.

2) Omega 3 fatty acids of fish oils can ward off allergies. It can be taken as fish or as supplements.

3) Allergic rhinitis has become a very common allergic problem, especially in Asia. Two important concepts we have to learn are :

a) A neglected sneeze leads to a wheeze. Hence treat rhinitis and prevent asthma.

b) Anti-leukatrienes are very good drugs. They are effective and also decrease the steroid load which will be there on patients if they consume steroid drugs.

17

SELF-TEST CHARTS

Is your cough allergic in nature ?

	Yes	No
1) Does the cough occur in a particular season or change of season ?	☐	☐
2) Is the cough aggravated in a particular season or change of season ?	☐	☐
3) Is it accompanied by bouts of sneezing as well ?	☐	☐
4) Is coughing more at night than during the daytime ?	☐	☐
5) Is there a history of bouts of sneezing, eczema, or coughing in the family, i.e., parents/siblings?	☐	☐
6) Did you have eczema in your childhood?	☐	☐

Interpretation—If the answer to even 2 of the above questions is Yes, the cough is allergic in nature.

Are the child's symptoms due to asthma ?

1) Has he frequent coughs ?	☐	☐
2) Has he frequent running nose ?	☐	☐
3) Does he get cough, sometimes followed by fever ?	☐	☐
4) Has he a wheeze in his chest ? (This can be ascertained by putting your ear against his chest).	☐	☐

Yes No

5) Has he or had he earlier oozing rash on his face ? ☐ ☐

6) Does he or did he get abdominal colic at any time ? ☐ ☐

Interpretation—The more 'Yes' he scores, the more likely he has asthma.

Is your child allergic to a food ?

Common Food Allergens

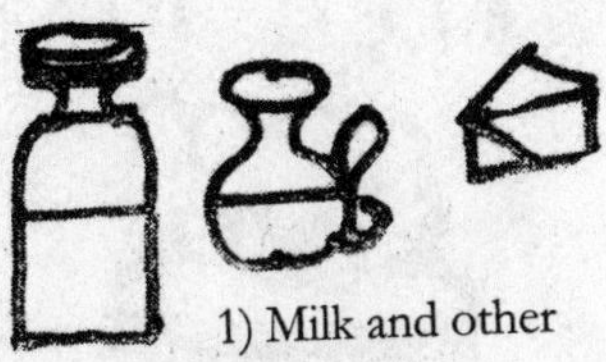

1) Milk and other diary products

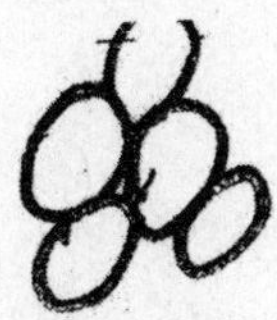

2) Eggs

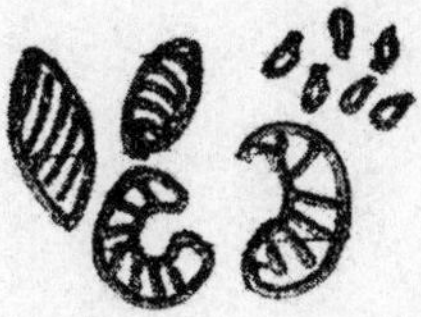

3) Nuts

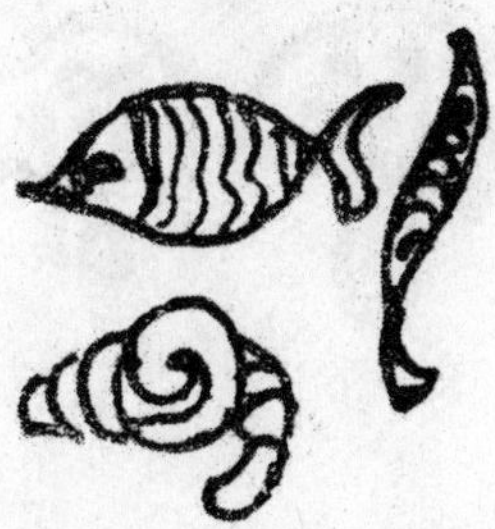

4) Fish

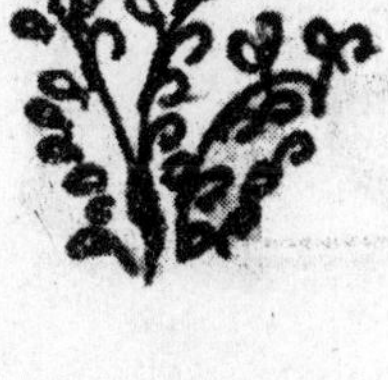

5) Wheat

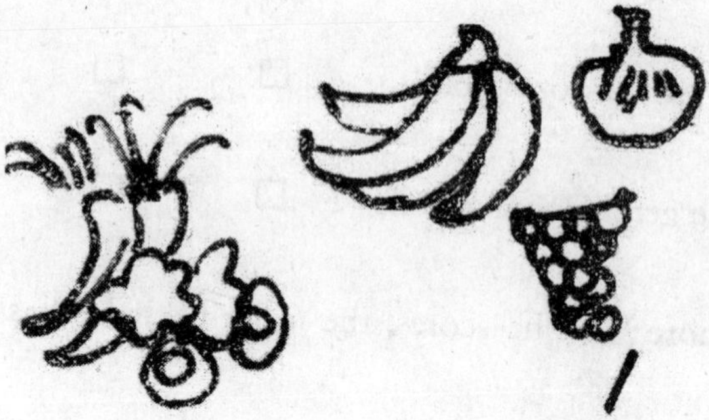

6) Fruits/Salads

7) Food additives

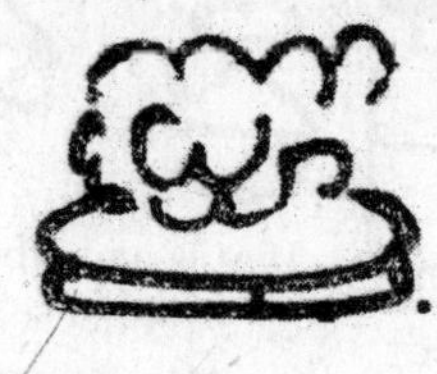

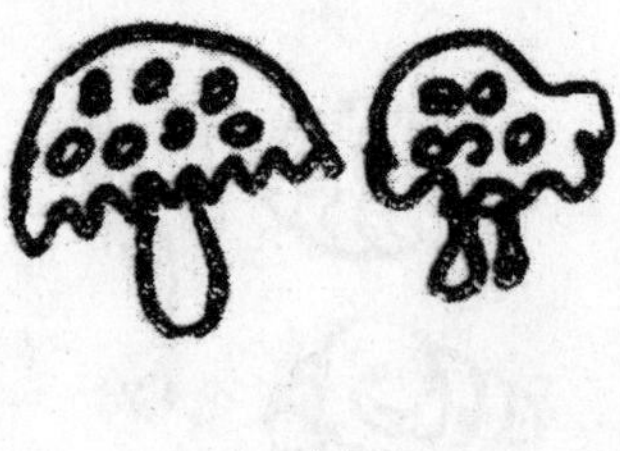

8) Mushrooms

9) Chocolates

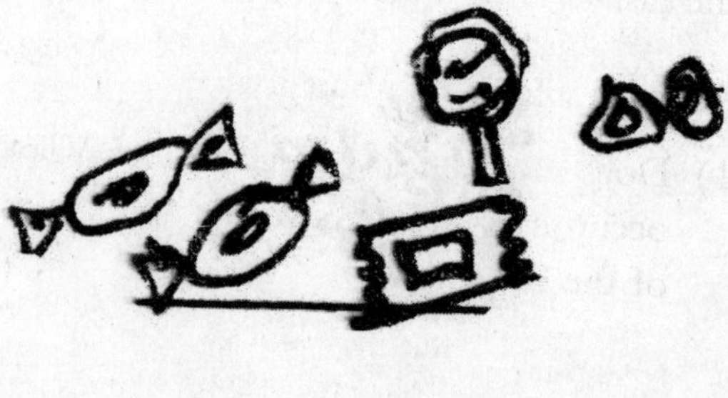

	Yes	No
1) Does he get rash around his lips and inside the mouth after taking a food ?	☐	☐
2) Does he vomit a particular food each time he takes it ?	☐	☐
3) Does he get abdominal colic ?	☐	☐
4) Is he losing weight because he cannot retain a particular essential food?	☐	☐
5) Has he a reddish oozing rash on his face?	☐	☐

Interpretation—The more the 'yes' answers, the more the chances of allergy to an article of food.

Is your skin rash allergic in nature ?

1) Does the rash appear and disappear repeatedly ?	☐	☐
2) Is the rash raised from the skin ?	☐	☐
3) Does it cause itching when it is there ?	☐	☐
4) Has the rash any relation to heat, cold, exertion, or emotional state ?	☐	☐
5) Does the rash appear after taking a particular food?	☐	☐

Interpretation—'Yes' to any of the above questions indicate that the rash is allergic in nature.

Are you allergic to hair dye ?

1) Does the need to scratch on the scalp occur after 24 hours of the application of the dye ?	☐	☐

2) Is there itching behind the ears and nape of the neck after 24 hours of the application ?	☐	☐
3) On examination is there redness and raised spots on the scalp ?	☐	☐

Interpretation—If the answer to any one question is 'Yes' you are allergic to that hairdye, and you must stop using it.

BIBLIOGRAPHY

Jaggi, Dr. O.P. *Asthma and Allergies*

Readers Digest, 'Is it harmful, Is it healthy?'

Peter Borrie, *Common Skin Diseases*

Guyton, *Textbook of Medical Physiology*

Robbins Pathlogic Basis of Disease

Paniker, C.K. Jayaram and R. Ananthanarayan, *Textbook of microbiology*

Indian Drug Reviews

Xavier, G.F. Raneis, *Yoga for Successful, Spiritual, Married and Student Life*

Studenikin M. and T. Sokolova, *Allergic Disorders in children*

Hope R.A. and J.M. Longmore, *Oxford Handbook of Clinical Medicine*

The Week supplements published by Jacob Mathew for Malayala Manorama Co. Ltd.

First Aid and Family Health, Blity Editions.

Rao V.A., *Textbook of Diseases of the Eye*

Satoskar, Kale, Bhandarkars *Pharmocology and Pharmacotherapeutics*

Nicholas Piramal's *Mediscan*, January 1999 Issue.

Brandwein Paul F., *Your Health and Safety*

Dr. Clifford Rose/Dr. Paul Davies, *Several Newspaper Columns: Answers to Migraine*

Medical journals and magazine strips.

Allergy—patient information booklet Kramer-Publication.

23.	Yoga Therapy	225/-
24.	Obesity	125/-
25.	Self Motivation	125/-
26.	Yoga for Health and Relaxation	95/-
27.	Women Disorders and Pregnancy	95/-
28.	A Guide to Body Pains	95/-
29.	Sex Education	95/-
30.	Common Diseases and Cure	95/-
31.	Pranayama for Better Life	95/-
32.	Herbal Home Remedies	95/-
33.	A Guide to Beauty and Skin Care	95/-
34.	A Guide to Heart Care	95/-
35.	A Guide to High Blood Pressure	90/-
36.	Cancer: Causes and Prevention	95/-
37.	Nature Cure for Common Diseases	95/-
38.	Good Health Through Food and Regimen	90/-
38.	A Guide to Allergies	125/-
40.	A Guide to Aging	95/-
41.	Ayurveda for Health & Beauty	95/-

Lotus PRESS

4263/3, Ansari Road,
Darya Ganj, New Delhi-110 002
Ph.: 32903912, 23280047,9811594448
E-mail: lotus_press@sify.com
www.lotuspress.co.in